Live Your Life

PAIN FREE

Medical Discoveries That Stop Chronic Pain

with John Stamatos, MD

and

Grace Forde, MD

Peter Kechejian, MD

Samuel Thampi, MD

Mary Milano Carter, APRN

2005

The Magni Company

McKinney, Texas 75070

ISBN   1-882330-54-4

Published by:
The Magni Company
PO Box 849
McKinney, Texas 75070
Email: *info@magnico.com*
Printed in the U.S.A.

Table of Contents

Introduction
John M. Stamatos, MD

In the past few years, the field of pain management has advanced considerably. With these new tools, most pain syndromes can be controlled, which allows patients to lead a relatively normal life. New miracle medications have been developed, specifically for pain management, and new procedures have made the treatment of pain much more precise. Patients no longer have to survive by the adage "just live with the pain."

The basics of pain management, however, have remained the same. The cornerstone of treatment is still a detailed evaluation by a pain management specialist, which includes a thorough physical examination. Once an appropriate diagnosis is determined, one of the new available tools can be used to treat the pain.

This book has a simple message. Life is too short to live with the pain. Pain is ignored and grossly under treated in this country. With this book, we hope to provide you with the knowledge necessary to talk to your health provider about your pain.

One common question is: Why is pain not treated well by health care providers? Mostly because there are too many barriers hindering adequate treatment, and health care providers are not effectively educated in the treatment of painful states. In general, a physician's training in pain management only occurs after they are already treating patients. Thus, it is not an official education but, instead, an informal on-the-job-training by other providers who are also unofficially trained. Nursing education is no better.

The general medical textbooks have revealed that, on average, less than a page of information is dedicated to pain management. Thus, the people responsible for the general care of patients are never really exposed to all the tools available for the treatment of pain. Unfortunately, without the education, health care providers are then reluctant to get involved with pain management. Compound that with the pressure on medicine to limit specialty care, the patient in pain is the one who loses in the long run.

From the patients' perspective, a visit to a primary care provider usually involves more problems than their time allows, consequently, pain is frequently ignored until it's out of control. Society also get involved with a "just say no to drugs" attitude. Thus, if a patient needs to take medications for pain, they are judged by family and friends.

A recent survey of pain patients reported that for every message the patient receives from a pain provider to take medication, they receive another eight messages from society to "just say no." Included in these statistics are all the well-known people who abuse the medications routinely used for the treatment of pain. Considering all this information, it is obvious why adequate pain management is difficult to achieve.

This book is designed to cover the major components of a multidisciplinary approach to the treatment of painful conditions. This is not the only way to treat pain, but it is one way to treat it, and we have used this method successfully to treat our patients. The book is divided into sections designed to explain the major components of pain management. Acute pain affects most people at some time in their life. Whether it's a broken bone or surgery, some form of pain control after the event is usually required. Understanding what to expect and what's available will help you navigate these episodes.

Chapter Seven, How to Talk to Your Doctor About Pain, covers various ways to describe your pain to your health care provider. As mentioned previously, precisely defining your pain helps providers offer the most appropriate care. This chapter also helps you better understand your pain, so that you can describe it better.

Chapter Four, Medications for Pain Management, reviews the medications that are available specifically for pain management, and the medications that are borrowed from other specialties. Why is this important—because, for example, the medication, mexilitine, is the drug of choice to treat the pain of diabetic neuropathy.

Chapter One, Interventional Pain Management, provides information on all existing and new procedures for pain management. The advantage to these procedures is that chronic pain management is not necessary. Once the problem is fixed, you can return to your life.

In Chapter Three, Neurological Approaches to Pain Management (Migraines), techniques outside the interventional pain process are discussed to treat other pain syndromes such as headaches, for example.

Once the pain is controlled, Chapter Five, Physical Therapy and Rehabilitation in Chronic Pain, examines the exercises required to maintain relief. Using a combination of all these pain management techniques should help you control your pain.

As the patient, you and your family are in the best position to manage and control your pain. We encourage you to use these tools wisely to obtain the best, appropriate care.

I believe that this book and these techniques can change your life!
John M. Stamatos, MD

Chapter One

Interventional Pain Management

John M. Stamatos, M.D.

John M. Stamatos, M.D. is the Medical Director of North American Partners in Pain Management and Plainview and Franklin Hospital Medical Center. He completed his medical training at the Uniformed Service University of Health Sciences and his residency in Anesthesiology and Pain Management at the Walter Reed Army Medical Center. A Diplomate of the American Board of Anesthesiology with the added qualification in Pain Management, Dr. Stamatos is also a licensed acupuncturist in the State of New York and is the author of the best selling book *Pain Buster*.

Interventional Pain

Interventional pain management is a distinct subsection of general pain management. Basically, if there is a single area causing the pain, the treatment should be focused on attacking that area rather than the whole body. Thus, in general, interventional pain specialists are trained in placing needles to specific areas of the body to treat problems.

The training of the interventionalists should include a significant amount of time learning the techniques of injection therapy for pain management. Training is usually a 1- to 2-year period of time where the provider is exposed to different types of procedures under the supervision of a pain specialist experienced in these techniques. When choosing a pain provider, it is important to ask about his or her training before any procedures are performed.

In most cases, these procedures are performed with the assistance of a fluoroscope or x-ray machine for precise placement of the injections. Since the basis of this therapy is to pinpoint the injection, exact localization of the needles is crucial for the success of the procedure; therefore, the radiologic guidance is important. With the use of a fluoroscope, the provider can visualize the bony structures of the body. With these landmarks, the expected location of nerves and other structures can be determined with accuracy. The fluoroscopic guidance cannot show the location of "non-bony structures," which are usually the target of the injection, but allows visualization of the needle tip in reference to the bones in the area.

In some cases, a Computerized Axial Tomography (CAT) scanner can also be used to localize the needle tips. The CAT scanner can show not only the position of bony structures, but also some soft tissues, thus, can provide very exact information as to the needle tip position. The disadvantages of using the CAT scanner include greatly increased time and cost of procedure. In most cases, the CAT scanner is really overkill for the accuracy needed for pain management procedures.

In a few instances, injections can be performed without the use of radiologic assistance. If the final position of the needle is not close to any bony landmarks such as with a trigger point injection into a muscle belly, the fluoroscope will not add to the accuracy of the injection. Also, a very small number of other procedures can be performed without radiologic guidance and should be performed at the discretion of the pain provider.

The basic philosophy of injection therapy is to get a small amount of medication very close to the area of injury to treat the problem. In general, the pain provider should target an area of inflammation where the localized inflammation is the source of the pain. Many areas of the body can have inflammatory response; muscles, joints, and nerves are most common areas that cause pain. Thus, they are the targets of interventional pain management.

Inflammation in a muscle is called a trigger point. It causes the muscle to spasm, and this spasm causes pain. Inflammation in a joint is usually called arthritis. With arthritis, any motion of that joint causes pain. Finally, inflammation of a nerve is called neuritis, and it is categorized as a sharp shooting pain. An example of neuritis is sciatica, where the pain shoots down an extremity in the distribution of the nerve.

Most of the time, the medication injected into these areas is a substance that reduces the inflammation causing the pain. The medication most commonly used is a steroid. Steroids are the most potent anti-inflammatory medication available. As described in the medication section of this book, no matter what tissue is inflamed, the steroid will actively reduce it. If the inflammation is gone, then, in most cases, so is the pain.

If the steroid is effective and reduces the swelling, as long as it does not return, the pain will stay away. In large doses, steroids can be detrimental to the body causing demineralization of bone and hormonal changes

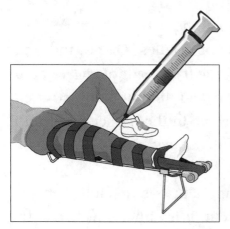

in general, but in the small doses needed for injection therapy, steroids have very little effect on the body as a whole. Thus, the injection of a steroid solution into an area of pain is the mainstay of interventional pain. A steroid injection into muscle is called a trigger point injection, into a joint is called a joint injection, and close to a nerve is called a nerve block.

If we cannot treat the inflammation, the other option available is to destroy the area with an ablative procedure. By destroying the area causing the discomfort, the source of the pain is removed. Ablative procedures can be performed by chemical agents, freezing the area (cryoablation), or burning the area (radiofrequency ablation). All of these techniques are discussed in greater detail later in this chapter.

Now that the rational behind interventional pain has been defined, I will describe the specific injections used in pain management. I'll start with the least invasive and end with the ablative techniques.

Acupuncture

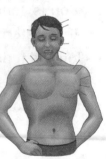

Though the philosophy of acupuncture is described later in the book, it is an interventional pain technique because it includes the use of needles. One of the techniques of acupuncture is the treatment of trigger point pain in muscles. This is called Ashi points, and it entails manipulating the needle in the trigger point until the irritation of the needle causes the spasms to release.

The advantage to acupuncture is no side effects or potential damage can occur. It is either effective in the treatment of the pain or there is no effect. Acupuncture needs to be performed in a series of sessions. Usually, there is a series of 10 sessions to get the pain under control, followed by maintenance treatments every week to a month to maintain the relief. Patients should start to feel relief from the treatments after the first three to four sessions. Acupuncture works well for disease states such as headaches and trigger points, but can also be used for just about any pain state.

Trigger Point Injections

As mentioned earlier, an injection into a spasmodic muscle is called a trigger point injection. The injectate itself can be many different solutions. Just manipulating the needle in the muscle can sometimes release the spasm; this is called dry needling. A local anesthetic injected into the muscle forces it to relax by causing paralysis of the spasmodic muscle. If a local anesthetic is used, its effect is short lived, 4 to 8 hours, but sometimes this period of relaxation forces the muscle to reset, and the spasm is released permanently. A combination of local anesthetic and steroid is the most common injectate for trigger point injections. With this combination, the muscle is forced to relax with the local anesthetic, and the steroid then reduces the inflammation, which can sometimes make the muscle relaxation last longer.

The basis of this therapy is to reset the muscle to act normally. We know that muscles have memory. That is how a golfer or baseball player can always move the club or bat the same way, even though it is moving so quickly. Once a muscle becomes spasmodic, the memory maintains the spasm, thus, the muscle thinks that this is its normal state. The trigger point injections try to re-educate the muscle to return to its normal non-spasmodic state. Once this is accomplished, the muscle should maintain that normal state.

Trigger point injections are usually given in series, with three to five areas injected during each session. The sessions should occur on a weekly or twice a week schedule to maintain the relief obtained with the injections. Multiple sessions can be used to treat the pain, and the injections should be continued as long as relief continues to improve. If the relief from the injections remains short lived after multiple sessions, then botox injections should be considered for more permanent relief. Syndromes that can be treated with trigger point injections include isolated muscle spasm, myofascial pain syndromes, and muscle fibrillations.

Joint Injection

Any joint in the body can become inflamed and cause pain. A steroid injection into a joint is a very common procedure to treat this pain. The irritation of the surface of the joint should be completely relieved with the steroid. On occasion, if the joint is very painful, a local anesthetic can be added to the injection. This will numb the area and reduce the pain for a short period of time.

If the steroid injection is effective, it can be repeated intermittently, as needed, without concern for bone breakdown. If the irritation is a result of the wearing down of the cartilage (osteoarthritis), in some joints such as the knees, an artificial cartilage-like material called hyaline can be injected into the joint to reduce the ongoing irritation in the joint. This material slowly wears down over time, but is effective in slowing down the ongoing deterioration of the joint. These injections can be repeated every 6 months to continue relief.

Any provider who is comfortable with this technique can perform joint injections. Providers should maintain records of each procedure and record how much steroid is injected into each joint to avoid adding too much steroid into any specific area of the body. As with most pain syndromes, once the area is adequately treated, physical therapy is essential to take advantage of the relief provided. The more the patient exercises with the joint treated, the less chance of requiring subsequent injections.

In addition to the joints in shoulders, knees, and hips where pain is obvious, lower back pain can come from small joints in the spine called the facet joints. These joints are on the side of the spine and located at every level of the spinal column. Normal activities of life cause arthritic changes in these joints. If the arthritis becomes

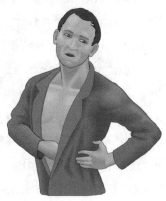

significant, the pain is localized to the lower back with minimal radiation into the legs past the knees.

The pain is spasmodic in nature and feels like a tightening across the lower back. Imaging studies of the lower back show the arthritic changes in the joints. Injections of steroids into these joints can significantly reduce the pain from this syndrome. Sometimes, there is pain from the facet joints and from herniated discs in the lower back. In that case, both areas should be injected to treat the pain.

Facet joint injections can be performed in any area of the spine and can be repeated every couple of months, as needed, to treat the pain. If the relief obtained from these injections is not prolonged, less then a couple of months, for example, then facet rhizotomy (described later in this chapter) can be used for longer periods of relief.

Nerve Blocks

This is a very broad term that applies to any injection placed in proximity to a nerve to try and reduce the irritation of a nerve. The most common nerve block is the epidural steroid injection. This injection is used to treat pain from irritation of a spinal nerve as they leave the spine. This is called radiculopathy, also known as sciatica, pain from herniated disc, or lumbago.

This pain radiates from the back down one or more extremity. It can also occur in the neck or the lower back. It usually comes from a herniated disc, a part of the spine that helps cushion the spine. If it is pushed out of place, it can hit a nerve, and that impact can cause pain in the nerve.

The other common cause is from a syndrome called spinal stenosis. This occurs when the canal where the spinal cord exists starts closing in on the spinal cord and that squeezing causes the pain. Spinal stenosis is a syndrome that takes many years to become symptomatic and is a progressive disease.

Post-laminectomy pain is another cause of radiculopathy. Sometimes after laminectomy or spinal fusion surgery, a significant amount of pain is still present. Evaluation by the surgeon concludes that the surgical repair is intact and does not need to be modified, but the patient still has a lot of pain. This can happen for a multitude of reasons, but the most common is scar tissue in the surgical areas irritating the nerves. Unfortunately, there is no surgical treatment for scar tissue and, thus, pain management techniques should be used to treat the pain. Other less common reasons for radicular pain include tumor growth into the spinal canal, fatty growth in the epidural space, and chemical irritation of the nerves called arachnoiditis.

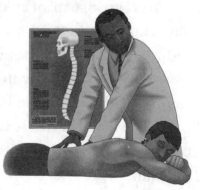

With an epidural steroid injection, a small amount of steroid is placed in a fat filled cavity around the nerve, called the epidural space, to reduce the irritation. Since the pain is from the irritation of the nerve, if the irritation is reduced, then the pain is also reduced. These injections can treat the pain. One of the common misconceptions of the injection is that it masks the pain rather than treating it. This is not true. The pain might return if the nerve becomes irritated again, but there is nothing in the injection to "numb" the pain, only treat it. This is one of the injections that should be performed with x-ray guidance to confirm that the injection is precisely near the area of nerve.

Multiple different approaches to the epidural space are available. An interventional pain provider can decide, with the patient, which approach is best for his or her specific pain syndrome. The two most common approaches are the translaminar approach with a midline approach and is used to treat bilateral pain. The other approach is the transforaminal approach and is used to treat pain that is predominantly on one side of the body. The injection can also be performed at all levels of the spine from the base of the neck to the bottom of the spinal canal.

The response to an epidural steroid injection is usually realized 2 to 3 days after the injection. If this procedure is expected to be successful, the patient should have 30 to 50% relief with a single injection. Injections can be repeated if there is progress in the relief of the pain. The usual series is three injections, and they can be repeated every 6 months, as needed, for control of the pain.

If there is no relief after the first injection, it is unlikely that subsequent injections will help reduce the pain. If there is no relief, the pain provider will probably consider another approach for the injection to obtain better relief. Take care; however, not to place too much steroid into the space because it can cause bone breakdown if used without discretion.

If performed correctly, the risks to the procedure should be minimal. Risks include failure to get the injection in the correct location, infection, bleeding, and nerve damage. These risks are minimized when the procedure is performed in an operating room or procedure area and x-ray guidance is used.

In addition to steroids, local anesthesia can be injected to anesthetize (numb) the nerve. This serves two purposes: 1) to reduce the pain of the nerve immediately, and 2) to determine if that is the source of the pain. If a surgeon is planning surgery and wants to determine which nerve or nerves is the source of the pain, this procedure can define the involved nerves.

Sometimes, concentrated salt water is also injected into the epidural space to reduce scar tissue; if, after spinal surgery, there is scar tissue tethering the nerve as it is leaving the spine. A very targeted injection of concentrated saline solution can help to breakdown the scar tissue and free up the nerve.

Another type of nerve block is a sympathetic nerve block. Some pain syndromes are a result of the sympathetic nervous system becoming irritated, and this creates pain. This disease state is called Complex Regional

Pain Syndrome (CRPS) and causes pain out of proportion to the injury that it is not consistent with the injury. One of the common symptoms of the disease is allodynia, which is pain to light touch. This means that the patient feels pain over the affected area, even if something just rubs up against the area. Local anesthetic injections into the area around the sympathetic nerves in the body are used to try and reset the nerves. This is the treatment of choice for this pain.

The sympathetic nerves for the upper extremities come together in the neck and are called the stellate ganglion. Injection of a local anesthetic into this area is called a stellate ganglion blockade. The injection is performed with x-ray guidance in a procedure area and should provide immediate relief of the symptoms.

In the lower extremity, the sympathetic nerves come together outside the bony spine in the lower back. The injection of local anesthetic to this area is called a lumbar sympathetic blockade. As with the stellate ganglion blockade, this injection is performed in a procedure area with x-ray guidance, and the relief should be immediate. If there is positive relief using these techniques, but the pain relief is not long-term, the procedure can be repeated to try and make the relief last longer.

Other nerve blocks include peripheral nerve blocks. These injections are performed when a nerve not in the spinal column becomes irritated. This can occur from trauma or surgery. If it occurs from a nerve trapped in scar tissue after surgery, then it is called a scar neuroma. Placing a small amount of steroid near the effected area should reduce the irritation and, hence, the pain. These injections can be repeated over time if the pain returns. If the pain continues to return, then nerve ablation can be considered as a more permanent solution.

Intercostal nerve blocks are used for patients with pain in the distribution of the intercostal nerve. Each rib has a nerve that courses on the bottom edge of the rib called the intercostal nerve. These nerves give us the strength of breathing in the rib cage. If there is pain in this area from a rib fracture or tumor growth into a rib, a knifelike pain that wraps around the chest wall into the middle of the chest occurs. This is called intercostal neuralgia. The pain is worse with motion of the chest wall and deep breathing. An intercostal nerve block is a procedure that places a small amount of local anesthetic and steroid close to this nerve. This stops the pain by treating the nerve. If the pain returns, the intercostal ablation can be considered.

Piriformis syndrome is when the piriformis muscle, which is deep inside the buttock, becomes spasmodic. The sciatic nerve passes through the muscle and can become irritated if the muscle is spasmodic. The diagnosis can be difficult because the pain from the piriformis muscle acts like lumbar radiculopathy. A steroid injection near the nerve should be effective to treat the irritation and reduce the pain.

When these therapies are effective, but don't provide long-term relief of pain, more advanced techniques of pain management can be used to try and lengthen the periods of relief that patients can have. The next section discusses the reversible procedures effective in reducing pain.

Nucleoplasty/Disc Decompression

Pain from a small-herniated disc (less than 6 mm) can be treated with this technique. Epidural steroid injections should be the first line treatment for this condition. If the relief from the injection does not last; however, nucleoplasty should be considered. Before performing this procedure, obtain a surgical consultation to confirm that the patient is a candidate.

This technique is performed as an outpatient procedure. It involves placing a needle into the middle of the herniated disc and extracting a small amount of the disc material. There are different ways to perform this extraction, but the procedure allows the disc material to be removed without surgery. The relief occurs within a few days after the procedure and should last as long as surgery because the offending disc is removed. Patients have limited activity over the next month to allow the disc to heal, but after that, patients should return to full activity.

Spinal Cord Stimulation

This is the use of electrical impulses in the epidural space to treat pain. The epidural space is the closest area to the spinal cord that we can safely access. As with the epidural steroid injections, we use this space for a multitude of pain management techniques.

With the spinal cord stimulator, electrodes are placed into the epidural space and can either be placed surgically through a small incision or through a needle. The electrodes are placed over the area where the nerves, in question, come into the spinal cord. For lower extremity pain, this location is usually in the thoracic spine or the midback area. Once the electrodes are in place, small impulses of electricity through the electrodes stimulate the spinal cord. This stimulation is like white noise to the brain.

The reason the stimulation works to treat the pain is still unknown. One way to describe the relief is that without the stimulation, 95% of the impulses going to the brain through the spinal cord are the pain. The stimulator creates impulses that the brain senses as a desirable tingling sensation. With the stimulator on, the tingling sensation overpowers the pain. Thus, that 95% of pain impulse going to the brain is reduced to 5% of the total input to the brain; the rest is the tingling sensation. Then the brain does not feel the pain but, instead, feels the tingling.

It can only control chronic pain. If an individual gets injured, he or she will still feel it the same as anyone

else. Even if another disc is herni-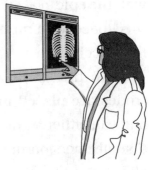
ated in the back, the stimulator
will not be able to treat it. The
brain can tell the difference between acute pain and chronic pain,
which follow different pathways in
the spinal cord; thus, acute pain
is not treated with spinal cord
stimulation.

A spinal cord stimulator, like most pain management procedures, is a relatively simple process to implant into the body. Though every pain specialist per-
forms this slightly different, there is a routine procedure to implant the device. The procedure is performed
in an operating room in a hospital or surgical center.

As with the epidural steroid injections, a needle is
placed into the epidural space and, through that
needle, an electrode is introduced into the epidural
space. With x-ray guidance, the electrode is moved to
the area over the spinal cord where stimulation is required. For most pain complaints, two electrodes
should be used to completely cover the areas of pain.
This part of the procedure is usually performed while
the patient is sedated.

At this point, the patient is awakened on the operating room table with the electrodes in place. The stimulator is turned on, and the patient is stimulated with
the electrodes. This part of the procedure is performed
to confirm that all of the areas of the patient's pain are
covered with the stimulation. If the areas are not, then

the electrodes can be moved to better cover the areas of pain.

Once the pain areas are covered with the stimulation, the patient is sedated again, and the electrodes are anchored into place under the skin, and tunneled out under the skin, to an area on the side of the body. The electrodes are then attached to a device that continues the stimulation. With this all in place, the patient is discharged to go home and test the stimulation. This period of time can vary from a couple of days to a couple of weeks and allows the patient to determine if the stimulation is effective in treating the pain.

If the stimulation controls the pain while the patient is performing his or her normal activities for the test period, then the stimulator is implanted; i.e., a small generator and battery is implanted to stimulate the electrodes on a permanent basis. If the electrodes do not provide adequate pain relief, the electrodes can be removed (explanted). One of the benefits of this device is that it is completely reversible. If there is not adequate stimulation, the electrodes are removed and no permanent changes are made to the body.

Once the stimulator is in place and working, the only maintenance for the device is to replace the battery source every couple of years, a minor surgical procedure. Unlike medications, the body cannot develop tolerance to the stimulation, thus, the relief of stimulation does not reduce over time.

This device is most commonly used for lumbar radiculopathy. Whether it is after spinal surgery and

there is still pain, even though the surgery was successful, or if there is significant pain from the spine,
and the patient is not a surgical candidate. It can be
used for pain from the lower back going into the legs or
from pain in the neck going into the arms. This device
can be used for other disease states such as complex
regional pain syndrome, peripheral vascular disease,
peripheral neuropathy, pelvic pain, urinary incontinence, and, most recently, for patients with chest pain
with no source. The same technology is used to treat
headaches and nerve injuries in the arms and legs.

Intrathecal Infusion Devices

This device is used to deliver medication into the
fluid around the spinal cord. We know that the recep-
tor in the body, placed where the medication works (for
narcotics and some antispasmodics), is in the spinal
cord. When patients take medication by mouth, the
medication goes into the stomach and is absorbed into
the bloodstream. The medication is then passed through
the liver and on to the rest of the body.

In the case of narcotics and antispasmodics, only a
small amount of oral medication gets to the spinal cord
to have its effect. Thus, patients must ingest a lot of
medication in order to have an effect. Also, when the
medication gets to the bloodstream, it travels through-
out the body. The amount that travels to the brain can
give the sedation and nausea associated with these medications. If the medication is delivered to the fluid around

the spinal cord, then it is being delivered directly to the area in the body where the receptors are located. This means that much less medication can be used to have the same effect.

In the case of narcotics, the factor is somewhere between 1 in 100 to 1000; i.e., 1 mg of morphine placed in this fluid provides the same amount of pain relief as 1000 mg of morphine taken orally. In addition, when the medication is delivered to this space, it does not travel to the rest of the body, so the side effects are much less. Anesthesiologists have used this space for years to deliver local anesthetic to the spine for surgery. This is called a spinal anesthetic.

Candidates for this procedure are patients who have failed conservative therapy; i.e., patients taking oral medication who are unable to get enough pain relief, or the side effects of the medications outweigh the benefits of the medications. When a patient has cancer and needs narcotic management for the pain, they are usually started on oral narcotics with the dose slowly increased over time.

Some patients have positive pain relief with minimal side effects, and this is ideal. Other patients; however, suffer increased side effects as the doses escalate and before they feel pain relief. These side effects can include sedation or constipation. When this happens, the side effects negate relief, the pain is still present, and the patient has further discomfort as a result of the side effects. This is unacceptable and these patients are candidates for this device.

Other patients that can benefit from this device are those individuals with pain that requires narcotic therapy, but even a small amount of narcotics cause a significant amount of side effects. These patients are also candidates for the infusion device.

Once a patient is identified as a candidate for the device, a test dose period is performed to confirm that the patient will obtain relief with the device. There are many ways to do this, but the general goal is to have the medication delivered to the fluid around the spinal cord, and the effects of the medication confirm that the pain is treated. Once it's established that the patient is responding to the medication, the device can be implanted.

This process is performed in an operating room. A catheter is inserted in the back into the space with the fluid called the intrathecal space. The catheter is then tunneled around, under the skin of the abdominal wall, next to the belly button. Next, a pump, the size of a hockey puck, is implanted to deliver the medication. This device holds a reservoir and drive mechanism that slowly delivers the inserted medication to the fluid around the spinal cord. Once the device is implanted, it will continue to deliver the medication to the intrathecal space and provide pain relief to the patient.

The medication in the device (and dose adjustments) can be handled and/or refilled in a simple office procedure, i.e., the fluid is removed and a new supply of medication is inserted. Typically, refills are necessary every 1 to 3 months, but the device itself, lasts 5 to 10 years, depending on use. As previously mentioned, an antispasmodic called Baclofen can also be administered through the device to control spasms from spinal cord injuries, multiple sclerosis, and/or brain injury.

When reversible procedures are ineffective in reducing pain, ablative procedures are available that destroy the structure in the body causing the pain. Although termed permanent blocks; the body usually regenerates the destroyed structure and the pain relief from these blocks only last about 4 to 6 months.

Botox Injections

In addition to its use as a wrinkle reduction technique, botox injections (botulism toxin) can be used to reduce muscle spasms that cannot be treated with trigger point injections. The botox is injected into the muscle belly, and it kills the muscle. Care is taken to only kill a small amount of muscle tissue. There is no decrease in muscle strength with these injections because such a small amount of muscle is destroyed. The muscle grows back over the course of time and, hopefully, when it grows back, it is not spasmodic and acts like normal muscle. Patients are candidates for this technique if they get excellent relief from the trigger point injections, but it is not long-term relief. The only risks to this procedure are if the botox kills the wrong tissue and/or it's injected into the wrong location. Select an appropriate, experienced provider to administer the injections to limit any potential problems.

Prolotherapy

This technique has been used since 1950 to treat painful states. The basis for this therapy is a presence of laxity in a ligament in the body that's causing pain. Forcing that ligament to contract down stops the laxity and treats the pain. Common areas where this occurs include the ankles, sacroiliac joints, and shoulders. In the ankles, it occurs in patients that constantly sprain their ankles, which causes the ligament to loosen up. If the ligament is loose, the ankle is at risk for repeat sprains.

In the sacroiliac joint, which is deep in the hip area, laxity can cause pain with motion. This joint is not supposed to have much motion, thus, the prolotherapy stops motion in the joint. In the shoulder, only the parts of the joint that are not supposed to move can be treated with prolotherapy.

This procedure is usually divided into a couple of sessions. An irritant medication is injected into the target area and can be accomplished without x-ray guidance in many cases. Once the medication is injected, there is usually a short time (a couple of weeks) of increased pain from the irritation.

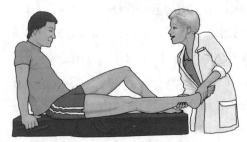

At the end of that time, once the amount of pain relief is established, the pain provider determines the number of subsequent injections that will be needed for the area. Once the ligament is tight, exercise is used to strengthen the muscle around the area so the pain does not return. The only risk of this procedure is if the medication is delivered to the wrong tissue. Injecting the wrong tissue can cause a pain syndrome in itself.

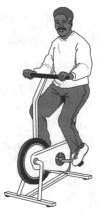

Radiofrequency Ablation

This technique uses a needle to deliver energy to the surrounding tissue to create heat. That heat destroys the tissue at the tip of the needle and leaves—what is best described as—a spot-weld mark where the tip of the needle was inserted, thus killing the tissue. It is called radiofrequency ablation because the heat is created by a very high-frequency output from the needle tip. The needle tip is the only place where the heat is generated, so only a discreet lesion (about 2 to 5 mm) is created by the procedure.

Radiofrequency ablation can be used for a multitude of areas in the body, but is commonly used for facet joint injections. With this outpatient procedure, the needles are placed in the correct position with x-ray guidance. The patient is then awakened and the needle tips are stimulated to determine their locations. Once confirmed (with this test) that the needles are in the correct position, the patient is re-sedated, and the ablative part of the procedure is performed.

Each lesion takes about 90 seconds to perform. After the procedure, it takes about 2 weeks to see the response of the ablation. If successful, the patient should get 4 to 6 months of relief from the procedure.

Intradiscal Electrothermocoagulation (IDET)

This is an extension of radiofrequency ablation. The difference is that this probe creates energy along its complete length instead of a small discreet lesion. Some pain from the spine occurs from the disc itself (called discogenic pain) and occurs when cracks form in the disc surface and the cushion material in the disc leaks out into the epidural space. The cracks are called fissures and the cushion material is called nucleus propulsus. The nucleus propulsus (NP) is extremely irritating to the spinal nerves and, when present in the epidural space, the irritation causes radicular-type pain, just like a herniated disc, but intermittent instead of constant. When some of the material is forced out, the pain occurs. If no NP is present, there is no pain.

To determine if a patient has discogenic pain, first perform a discogram (described earlier). This procedure allows interventional pain specialists to determine if any fissures are present in the disc. If so, the patient is a candidate for the Intradiscal Electrothermal Annuloplasty (IDET). Before IDET, the only treatment available for discogenic pain was fusion of the disc space. With IDET, a needle is placed into the disc. and a wire is slowly advanced around the wall of the disc where the fissure is located. This is performed with x-ray guidance.

Once the wire is through the area with the fissure, the radiofrequency technique is used to heat the wall of the disc and seal the fissure. The heating can take up to 20 minutes to completely seal the fissure. Once the fissure is closed, there should be no further leakage. Once the procedure is complete, it takes a couple of weeks for the pain to resolve completely. At that point, the patient can return to a normal activity level with increasing exercise.

Cryoablation

This procedure is almost the opposite of radiofrequency ablation. Instead of heat to kill, cryoablation uses cold to freeze tissue. Also a needle technique, once the needle is placed appropriately, liquid nitrous oxide is passed through it. Using a refrigeration process, the tip of the needle reaches temperature of -70 degrees Celsius. Anything created in the ice ball is killed. One of the advantages to this procedure is that although the tissue is killed, it can grow back more easily than with other destructive lesions, so it is considered a gentler way to kill tissue. As with the radiofrequency ablation, the risk in this procedure is to confirm that the correct tissue is killed and not to damage unnecessary tissue.

Chemical Ablation

The final neuroablative techniques available are alcohol or phenol ablative techniques. If a larger area needs to be destroyed, dehydrated alcohol or phenol can be injected to destroy the tissue. The lesion created is not as precise, as with the other techniques, and there is no way to control the spread of the lesion, but depending on what needs to be killed, this can be the technique of choice.

Many areas of pain can be controlled with these neuroablative techniques.

Intercostal Neuroablation

As described above, if intercostals nerve blocks work to control the pain from the intercostal nerve, but do not last long enough, consider ablation to provide the area with 4 to 6 months of relief.

Celiac Plexus Ablation

For patients with pancreatic cancer, there is a deep aching discomfort in the abdomen that is very difficult to treat with medication. The pain can be so bad, the patient is unable to eat, which adds to the patient's suffering. The celiac plexus is the group of nerves that serves the area of this pain. A celiac plexus ablation, or destroying these nerves, can give the patient 4 to 6 months of relief without having to use any medications at all. It provides these terminally ill patients a better quality of life until their demise.

Superior Hypogastric Plexus Ablation

This group of nerves serves the pelvic area, thus, patients with cancer growth causing pain in the pelvic area can be treated with this technique.

Conclusion

There are very few areas in the body where interventional pain techniques cannot be used to treat pain. This chapter provides an overview of multiple, different techniques that can be used. As with any medical condition, the most important function of care is to determine what's best for each patient and individualize each treatment plan. Thus, each specific case should be discussed with the pain provider to determine the best way to treat the individual condition. Also, it is important to remember to try and treat all pain syndromes with reversible techniques but, if necessary, ablative techniques can be used to give longer-term relief.

Notes

Chapter Two

What to Expect From Acute Pain Management

Peter A. Kechejian, M.D.

Peter A. Kechejian, M.D. is an Interventional Pain Specialist and Director of Oncology Pain Services for North American Partners in Pain Management. A graduate of Georgetown School of Medicine, he completed his residency in Anesthesiology and fellowship in Pain Management at the University of Massachusetts Medical Center. Dr. Kechejian is a diplomate of the American Board of Anesthesiology with a Subspecialty Certification in Pain Management. He is formerly the Director of the Anesthesiology Pain Management Program at the Nassau University Medical Center on Long Island. He is a member of the International Spinal Injection Society and The New York State Society of Anesthesiologists.

What to Expect From Acute Pain Management

Introduction

To the millions of acute pain sufferers in this country and in the world, there is hope of obtaining relief and avoiding unnecessary suffering after operative procedures and severe accidents causing trauma. We will limit this discussion of acute pain management to hospital-based care since most of the outpatient, acute care is treated by a patient's primary care physician. With the advancement of pain management in the hospital setting, particularly in the United States, more aggressive technologies beyond oral medications and intramuscular injections are now becoming more readily available. Intravenous patient-controlled analgesia (IV-PCA) narcotic pump therapies and epidural catheter techniques are two advanced pain management strategies that control pain beyond the use of oral pain medications alone. In addition, anesthesiologists in this country have been primarily responsible for the advancement of regional anesthetic techniques such as nerve blocks, before and after surgeries, to treat patients with acute pain.

Patients need not worry excessively about enduring severe postoperative pain if, after major operations,

physicians recognize that, along with their other disease processes, patients will experience pain that requires primary medical attention. If a patient comes
into a hospital for an appendectomy, for example, he/
she can expect at least a day or two of moderate—or
even an element of severe—pain, and then expect, with
further healing, that this pain will start to lessen and
be more controllable. Likewise, after a major automo-
bile accident (acute trauma pain) that may cause a bony
fracture type of pain, a patient will initially feel moderate to severe pain intensity and then, with further healing, they can expect less pain intensity as they move
into a rehabilitative phase of care.

No matter what the cause or intensity of the pain, it
can certainly be treated to the extent of known medical
science, a body of knowledge that grows every year. Patients need to realize that pain specialists are available
to help them along the way depending how they heal.

Historically, postoperative pain relief was administered mostly using oral or injectable narcotics for a
period of time, but this was not working for the major-

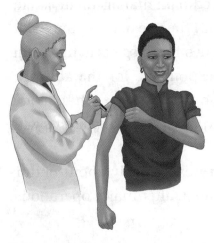

ity of patients. One of the
problems was that these
narcotics were given on an
as-needed basis when, in
fact, patients were hurting
all of the time after major
operations. Frequently,
their pain was under
treated. With more patient

pain complaints and other kinds of acute pain processes that led to a chronic pain process, physicians recognized the need to involve pain specialists to try and help patients in a more comprehensive way. Getting better control of their pain symptoms earlier in the care process ultimately led to better outcomes in the long run.

Many hospitals have an acute pain management service, typically run by the anesthesiology department, where physicians can consult with pain specialists to better care for their patients. Beyond this is the specialty-trained pain management doctor who can provide a more comprehensive evaluation and treatment plan, as necessary.

Extent of the Problem

Literally hundreds of thousands of operations are performed on a yearly basis and, unfortunately, thousands of major accidents—either from motor vehicle accidents or work related causes—result in a tremendous amount of acute pain. Ongoing pain research revealed that intense acute pain could lead to a more chronic process if not aggressively controlled. This realization motivated physicians to treat severe pain more seriously. It appears that more aggressive treatment of the acute phase of injury can help gain better control of a patient's symptoms and lead to a better rehabilitative outcome.

Evidence exists that uncontrollable acute pain can change the nervous system and the way pain travels in the body. These changing processes lead to a more chronic pain process. Longer-term pain conditions can be of various types and are typically more difficult to control, compared to the original pain. Look at the amount of disability in this country; it's a huge issue. Not only the cost to the patient from loss of work, pain, and suffering, but also as a nation from loss workdays and productivity.

It is the persistent high intensity and frequency of pain in all these patients, and the overburdening nature of chronic pain care on primary care doctors, that led this nation to develop a pain management specialty in medicine. There was, essentially, an outcry for improvement in pain management, both at the patient level and, also, at the regulatory levels such as the Joint Commission of Accreditation of Hospitals. In the last 10 years, particularly, pain management has made great strides to help patients, both in the outpatient setting and in the hospital setting, with their various pain management needs.

Who Is at Risk?

Virtually, every patient is at risk for developing an acute pain state, but particular attention is given to the very young and the very old patient population. These patients tend to be under assessed, or it was assumed that they, perhaps, do not experience as much pain as young or middle-aged adults. It was once thought that babies, when they were born, were incapable of developing acute pain because their nervous systems were underdeveloped. This was later disproved and, in fact, we now know that infants have a fully developed pain management nervous system and are quite capable of feeling pain at birth.

Older patients, for whatever reasons (perhaps dementia or an inability to communicate), are often disregarded and physicians assumed that they did not experience as much pain. Older patients may view pain management as a normal process of aging and dying. These views certainly do not need to be accepted, and pain management specialists are continuing their efforts to educate the public regarding all types of pain, in all age groups, and how it can be managed more effectively than in the past.

More aggressive operations or more severe accidents can be expected to cause more severe pain, both in the acute phase and into the rehabilitative phase. Awareness of this, at the patient and physician level, should translate to better pain management care in the short and the long run.

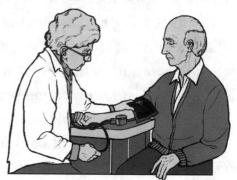

Assessment

There are various ways to assess pain in patients. Although there may be no true objective way, a patient report of pain using a verbal pain score is considered the gold standard of pain evaluation. Pain can be rated in intensity using a "0 to 10" rating scale, where "0" (zero) is no pain and "10" is the worst pain you can imagine. This scale works well in adults and older children. In younger children, who do not understand a 0 to 10-pain scale, a "facial" pain scale can be used, depicting a "sad, crying" face on one side of the scale and a "happy, smiling" face on the other side. Younger children, perhaps up to the age of 7 years old, do very well with this pain assessment scale. Elderly patients, who may have dementia or are less communicative, can best be assessed by an objective behavior scale, that is, observing grimacing, pain behavior, and vital signs such as blood pressure and heart rate, for example.

One of the key factors that pain management specialists understand, perhaps better than anyone, is to believe their patients—based on their pain score—not only subjectively, but also combining objective findings when examining patients. Patients need to feel believed when they report pain to their nurses or doctors. Honest and open communication between both patient and physician typically leads to more effective pain control.

Proper assessment of pain in patients involves not only doing an initial evaluation and treatment plan, but also having patients reassessed frequently based on the severity of their pain. To ensure this assessment, as treatment progresses, patients are best taken care of based on the changing nature of their pain. For example, if the patient has a motor vehicle accident and ruptures his or her spleen, and, subsequently, undergoes a major operation to remove the spleen to control the hemorrhage, these patients may be given intravenous narcotics such as morphine every three hours, around-the-clock, in an attempt to control their acute postoperative pain. If patients are still complaining of high pain, say "7/10" or more on the verbal pain scale, consider increasing the individual dose of morphine to provide more comfort, provided their vital signs are stable. If patients are over sedated, attempt to lower the dose or space the injections less frequently, but still provide enough primary pain relief. At any rate, frequent assessments of pain help guide the treating doctors to effect the necessary changes in pain care plan.

Diagnosis of Various Pain Types

The majority of patients who suffer from traumatic and postoperative pain typically have a musculoskeletal type of injury that causes the pain they experience. Soft tissues such as muscle and skin are irritated, or bones that are fractured, give the patient a certain pain sensation that is more readily controllable, compared to specific nerve injury. Nerve pain is typically more difficult to control than soft tissue or bone pain because it can be more resistant to traditional medication treatment. A certain level of morphine narcotic therapy, for example, may help patients with shoulder muscle or bone pain, but do very little to help a shoulder nerve injury.

Typically, it would take twice or even more morphine, in this case, before the nerve injury component of pain feels improved. Patients who have injuries to their major organs, either in their chest or abdomen, also have a certain type of pain that is typically controllable—if not with anti-inflammatory medications, then with stronger and stronger narcotic medications. Psychological factors can play a role in a patient's overall pain man-

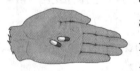

agement such as excessive anxiety and depression and can make treatment a little more difficult if these issues are not addressed.

Patients who have experienced acute appendicitis may recall that part of the pain they felt was in their abdomen, particularly on the right lower side, which occurs when the appendix is inflamed. If they had the operation, they remember that they hurt postoperatively in both the incision area and deeper in the belly. This type of pain is typically controlled with an anti-inflammatory medication, either orally or injectable. In many cases, a narcotic medication in either oral or injectable form is dosed to control the acute postoperative phase.

The patient should communicate to his or her nurses and physicians how the pain is being controlled and if any excessive side effects are intervening such as nausea, vomiting, constipation, itchiness, or over sedation. These types of side effects are typical when narcotics are used.

Potential nerve injury is a type of pain that is typically more difficult to control, short term and long term. Nerve pain does not usually respond to the traditional anti-inflammatory or narcotic type medication approach, but, rather, to a variety of different anti-nerve medications that have been used by pain specialists through the years. These medications are used in an attempt to quiet down nerve endings. The importance of involving a pain specialist, especially if pain becomes intractable or continues to persist, is to try and tease out these different types of pain and direct medications more specifically and comprehensively. This gives the patient a better relief outcome and moves forward with their care.

Treatment Options

Traditionally, oral and injectable narcotic medications have been used for acute pain management, along with adjuvant medications such as steroids, muscle relaxants, or anti-nerve agents. These medications are used in both an outpatient and inpatient setting. More often now, hospital-based pain care involves the use of intravenous patient-controlled analgesia morphine pumps, especially in the severe pain setting. The use of an intravenous line allows patients to give themselves small amounts of narcotic through a bedside pump, in shorter time intervals, to better control their pain.

These patient-controlled pain pumps are preferred over the traditional approach of communicating to nurses to draw up and administer the narcotics intramuscularly. Nurses typically have several patients on their shift that demand more time, which delays patients receiving their pain medication in a timely fashion. The intramuscular method of narcotic administration hurts with injection and can take a variable amount of time to reach its full effect, but using a pain pump avoids the need to call a nurse, and patients have a much shorter waiting period before the pain improves. Patients tend to use less narcotic, have fewer side effects, and are more comfortable while using the pain pump.

Intravenous narcotic pumps are typically set by specialists in the hospital and can be adjusted, based on patient's need and any other intervening side effects. Pumps are set at various intervals, so patients need to wait a specified amount of time before they can administer an additional dose. This so-called "delay time" between doses is for safety reasons and is designed to prevent patients from overdose problems. Typically, a 6 to 10 minute delay time between injections is normal, to allow the individual injection enough time to have its effect. Patients can push the narcotic button once, twice, or three times an hour to maintain their comfort, and this seems to work better than having larger amounts injected intramuscularly every 2, 3, or 4 hours, as an alternative route.

With the pumps, patients tend to have fewer side effects such as nausea, vomiting, or over sedation and have better pain scores, as mentioned previously. These intravenous pumps can, in certain circumstances, be programmed to give patients hourly amounts of narcotic, in addition to the doses the patient draws from the pump. These continuous narcotic rates are considered in settings where patients' narcotic requirements are typically high because they were previously on narcotics and are tolerant, or their pain is of an extreme, severe, and continuous nature.

Epidural catheter techniques have become more popular in hospitals for acute and post-traumatic pain, where local anesthetic and narcotic is administered in the spinal space. These spinal catheters are used as a more aggressive method to control pain, especially if other medical pain management methods are failing.

The most popular use of epidural techniques is for women in labor delivering babies, so they do not experience the severe pain of childbirth. Not every patient is considered a candidate for an epidural catheter, but in circumstances where it applies, it is considered one of the best methods to control pain. There are certain regions of the body where epidural catheter techniques work best. Major chest and abdominal operations or trauma to the legs are best suited for epidural techniques.

Deciding on a treatment option is individual, depending on several factors involved in an evaluation, especially a patient's age. A 3-year-old patient, after a major operation, is not a candidate for an intravenous narcotic pump, since he or she does not understand how it works. A patient's co-existing diseases would also make a difference in treatment options, as would the stability of their vital signs, particularly in trauma patients in an intensive care unit setting. For example, an intravenous narcotic self-controlled pump would not be a treatment option for a patient in a coma.

The extent of patient injury, particularly where the pain generator locations are, also makes a difference in treatment options. If a patient hurts from head to toe, just blocking the patient's legs with an epidural pain catheter technique, for example, would be inadequate as a treatment in and of itself, as opposed to using an oral or intravenous medication such as intravenous morphine, which covers all pain areas in the body.

Expectations of how long a particular type of pain should last are also factored into various acute pain management options. Again, the example of having an appendix surgery; a patient is expected to have pain for about a week's time and, then, recover fully. A patient who has fractured several bones, however, can be expected to hurt not only acutely, but also during the rehabilitative phase. In this case, pain management needs to continue into the rehabilitative phase to ensure that these patients are adequately covered as they move forward with their care.

Prescribed Treatment Plans

Typically, a patient's physician, who is caring for them, such as his or her surgeon or primary care doctor, will prescribe initial pain management medications and therapy for moderate to severe pain. This is generally by way of an intravenous route (hospital setting) or an oral pain medication route (both hospital and at home setting). If patients are not doing well or need a specialty consultation, they are encouraged to ask their physicians for a pain management specialty consultation, which offers a more comprehensive evaluation and adjustment in their pain medications. Many physicians in hospitals are amenable to consultation, particularly if they feel the patient's pain is not adequately controlled.

A patient taking Percocet, for example, or even a patient using intravenous morphine who is not controlled, may be a candidate for a day or two of intravenous, self-controlled, narcotic pump therapy, as previously described. The narcotic intravenous pump may be required to get their pain under better control, whereas other methods have failed to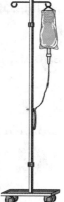

provide adequate relief. It seems apparent that when patients use this technology, they can self-administer to the effective comfort level better than any other source of treatment. If they are comfortable, they will not use the narcotic button and only take the doses they need for different times when they have pain, particularly with activity. Pain is expected to be less when they are at rest and to increase with activity.

With continued healing and reductions in the intensity of pain, patients need to know when the intravenous pain pump will be discontinued. Typically, patients are switched to oral narcotic pain medications when they can tolerate a liquid or solid diet, when their intravenous narcotic usage can be switched to an equivalent oral narcotic dosing, and when they are nearing discharge from the hospital. With any prescribed treatment plan, reassessment is always the critical factor, looking for the degree of desired comfort and any intervening side effects.

Many patients, after surgeries or trauma, are given a regional anesthetic, either by the surgeon or the anesthesiologist taking care of the patient. In an acute pain

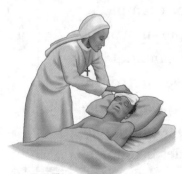

setting, a regional anesthetic is a local anesthesia injection at or around the painful site or directed around particular nerves that control pain sensation to an area. This can be quite helpful for controlling intense pain. Patients who go to a dentist, for example, know very well that local anesthetic injections for filling cavities can make a big difference in comfort. Likewise, if patients have had a major knee operation, injecting local anesthetic around the nerves in the leg can help with comfort by providing a numbing sensation, so they do not feel the high intensity of pain. Many times when these injections wear off, the pain increases, but this is typically managed more effectively with anti-inflammatory and narcotic medications.

Case Example

A 50-year-old gentleman is involved in a motor vehicle accident suffering multiple rib fractures and lung collapse. He has a previous history of chronic obstructive pulmonary disease and has been a two pack-a-day smoker. He comes into the hospital with severe pain and difficulty breathing. He is given intravenous narcotics, but this is not controlling his pain adequately, and he is getting over sedated. He is in intensive care and the intensivist calls for a pain management consultation, asking for an epidural catheter technique to control this patient's pain more effectively.

After a discussion with the patient, the epidural catheter is placed in the thoracic spine and local anesthetic and low dose narcotic is administered. The patient gets relief from "7/10 to 8/10" pain, down to "2/10" pain on the verbal pain scale and is breathing more effectively.

He is also better able to cough, which clears lung secretions helping to avoid the possible complications of pneumonia. The patient keeps this epidural catheter for 3 days, and then it is removed, and he is placed on oral Percocet for further pain relief, as he continues to heal his fractures. He had a severe coughing fit, which increased his pain to "9/10" for which he was given an intravenous patient-controlled morphine pump. After self-medicating, his pain decreased to a "2/10" level. He kept the IV-PCA for 2 days after which he resumed taking the Percocet, as needed. At discharge, the patient was given a prescription of Percocet for a week before follow-up with his physician.

This case example illustrates several important points about acute pain management in the trauma setting. The patient is assessed and given the best means of pain management to control his symptoms with the fewest side effects. Initially, intravenous narcotic was not effective, so an epidural catheter got this patient's rib fracture pain under control. Epidural catheters can stay in place for only a short while, so it was removed after 3 days to minimize risk of infection.

The patient tried to go directly to an oral narcotic, but was having increased pain; therefore, he was given the intravenous narcotic pump to self-dose for better comfort for a few days. After the intravenous self-controlled pump, the patient was able to transition to an oral narcotic; both at the end of his hospital stay and into his rehabilitative outpatient care. Aggressive attention to this patient's changing pain management needs carried him through a difficult period in his life, a period that could have ended his life had he not received the kind of pain care necessary to keep his breathing and lung function optimal.

Case Example

A 65-year-old female came into the hospital with a history of small bowel obstruction and "10/10" pain in her abdomen. She was previously taking six Percocets a day, at home, for chronic back pain. After a thorough workup, she was taken to the operating room where her surgeon removed a portion of diseased bowel. In the recovery room, she had "7/10" pain and was given a total of 15 milligrams of morphine. She had previously received 10 milligrams of morphine just prior to leaving the operating room. Her abdominal pain decreased to "4/10" and she was started on a patient-controlled morphine pump after receiving instructions regarding its use.

While the patient was on the surgical floor, she required frequent adjustments in her morphine dosage. At one point, she became nauseated and was evaluated by her surgical team. After concluding that there were no complications postoperatively to explain the nausea, it was determined that the patient was nauseated from the high usage on the morphine pump. The patient was subsequently given anti-nausea medication and she improved greatly. After the fourth postoperative day, bowel function returned and the patient's pain was averaging around "3/10 to 5/10." She was taking fluids well without nausea and was taken off the morphine pump. In its place, the patient was started on Vicoden (hydrocodone/tylenol oral medication combination) and Vioxx (an oral anti-inflammatory medication). She continued to have her pain well controlled and was discharged from the hospital the next day.

This case example, like the previous one, illustrates several important acute pain management principles in a postoperative patient. Major abdominal operations typically result in a moderate to severe pain state that necessitates a postoperative pain plan to rapidly meet changing pain intensities. By virtue of this patient already on Percocet prior to admission, she was quite tolerant to narcotics and would need very high doses of postoperative narcotic to control her pain. A patient-controlled morphine pump was started immediately, postoperatively, to treat her severe pain. The patient was doing well until she became nauseated, which was treated with relief.

Intervening side effects such as nausea should be rapidly recognized and treated for patient comfort, while continuing to treat the primary pain problem. The patient, fortunately, continued to progress well, and when bowel function returned, the patient was started on two oral pain medications. One of these medications was Vioxx, an anti-inflammatory medication that doesn't affect platelet and bleeding function. It is not typically strong enough to control postoperative alone, so it was combined with Vicoden oral narcotic.

When anti-inflammatory and narcotic medications are used together, they have additive pain relief effects that work much better than just using either Vioxx or Vicoden alone. If this patient had developed a more complicated postoperative course with frequent severe flares of intense pain, then, perhaps, a pain specialist consultation would have been called by the surgical team to better manage and restore this patient's comfort. In this case, epidural catheter, local anesthetic, continuous infusion would have been an advanced pain-care option until further progression of postoperative healing.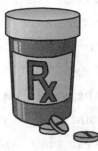

Conclusion

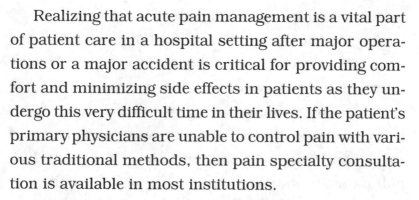

Realizing that acute pain management is a vital part of patient care in a hospital setting after major operations or a major accident is critical for providing comfort and minimizing side effects in patients as they undergo this very difficult time in their lives. If the patient's primary physicians are unable to control pain with various traditional methods, then pain specialty consultation is available in most institutions.

The focus of this chapter is acute pain in a hospital setting; however, this also applies to outpatient settings where patients experience acute pain, but do not need hospitalizations. The patients in the outpatient setting typically try over-the-counter medications or prescriptions given by their primary physicians such as anti-inflammatory medications and oral narcotics. This strategy typically works for the majority of patients. There are still a number of patients, however, who need emergency room evaluation for their ongoing pain and, invariably, several of these patients are admitted to the hospital for more aggressive care, as previously outlined in this chapter.

One of the key factors to keep in mind is when acute pain is better controlled; it tends to not leave the patients experiencing a more chronic, exacerbated pain state as they heal. If one type of pain management technique is not working, then another technique needs to be used until the pain is better controlled. Above all, the comfort and safety of the patient is the most important goal as an acute pain state is managed, and this care plan works best when left in the hands of trained pain management professionals.

As previously mentioned, although most of the acute pain management in hospitals is covered by the anesthesiology service, it is the preexisting chronic pain patient—who suffers from an acute injury or from severe postoperative pain—who is at increased risk of suffering with pain and one of the most difficult pain situations to control. This is where the real expertise of the pain management specialist shines through, typically "saving the day" for all those involved with trying to manage the chronic pain patient's "new" pain.

These chronic pain patients should never hesitate to ask their treating physicians for a pain management consultation, especially if they feel their pain is not adequately controlled. A pain specialist is best at not only understanding a preexisting pain state (as many pain specialty practices treat these conditions on a daily basis in the outpatient setting), but also determining what the patient has been through and where he or she needs to be in order to achieve improved comfort and move forward.

These chronic pain patients should not fear being labeled as drug abusers or addicts because their narcotic requirements are so high. It is just a fact of life that they are so tolerant to narcotic treatment effects (both to the pain relief effects and to the potential side effects). This tolerance needs to be recognized and adequate doses of pain medications need to be administered. Perhaps total pain relief is not practical in these situations, but keeping patients out of "intractable" pain should be a realistic end point.

Whatever situation patients find themselves in that involves acute, severe pain, this agony should be treated as an emergency and deserves the most aggressive pain care evaluation and treatment possible, so these patients can, eventually, feel better and continue to live their lives. This philosophy of pain care needs to be shared by everyone.

Notes

Chapter Three
Back & Neck Pain

John M. Stamatos, M.D.

John M. Stamatos, M.D. is the Director of Pain Management at North American Partners in Pain Management and Plainview and Franklin Hospital Medical Center. He completed his medical training at the Uniformed Service University of Health Sciences and his residency in Anesthesiology and Pain Management at the Walter Reed Army Medical Center. A Diplomate of the American Board of Anesthesiology with the added qualification in Pain Management, Dr. Stamatos is also a licensed acupuncturist in the State of New York and is the author of the best selling book *Pain Buster*.

Back & Neck Pain

Back and neck pain comprise the majority of lost workdays in the United states. It is rare for individuals not to succumb to this type of pain sometime in their life. Many various disorders can cause this type of pain and determining the exact source of the pain makes treatment that much easier.

Describe the Pain

The first step in describing back pain is to divide it into radiating or nonradiating pain; for example, if the pain stays in the lower back and buttocks, it's non-radiating; if it goes down the legs, it's radiating. We call pain that remains in the back, axial pain, and pain that radiates into the legs, radicular pain. Pain that radiates into the legs is usually caused by the irritation of a spinal nerve. When the nerve is irritated, the pain is felt along the path of the nerve; thus, an irritated spinal nerve in the lower spine causes pain to go down the leg or both legs. The pain is sharp, in nature, and usually has a shooting component.

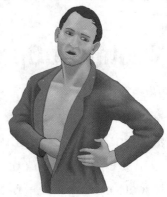

The nerve most commonly becomes irritated because of a

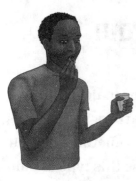

disc banging into it. This is called a herniated disc or sciatica. A disc can herniate from a multitude of reasons; for example, from a traumatic injury to an area to a twisting incident of the lower back. You can tell which nerve is involved by where the pain is located. If more than one nerve is involved, the pain follows all the affected nerves. When the nerve root becomes irritated, it swells. The pain that patients feel is directly related to the amount of swelling that is present and, as long as the nerve is swollen, there is pain. The herniation usually does not continue to press in the nerve but, in fact, once it has injured the nerve, it will pull back to a more normal position. The pain is not because of the herniated disc, but because of the swelling of the nerve root.

In a lot of cases, the nerve is injured, swells, and then heals itself in a couple of days; thus, the pain resolves without any care. If it does not get better on its own, then active treatment is necessary to correct the problem.

Treatment Options

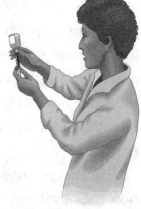

The first step for treatment is an oral anti-inflammatory. If this is ineffective, then epidural steroid injections are the next course of action. Other treatments to consider, if the epidural steroid is ineffective to give long-term relief, are spinal cord stimulation or nucleoplasty. These are described in Chapter One: Interventional Pain Management.

Once the swelling of the nerve is under control, the pain decreases, but this is only part of the battle. The herniated disc is still present and will cause pain again if something is not done to protect the area. Once the swelling of the nerve is reduced and the pain is better, patients must make an effort to strengthen their backs to prevent reinjury to the nerve. This is where physical therapy is essential. Without exercise, the area is left vulnerable and can be easily reinjuried. Once the muscles are strong enough around the area, the body can heal the disc, over time, so it cannot injure the nerve again.

Surgery

Surgical intervention for this problem should only be considered if the pain continues, despite these treatments, in the presence of weakness in the leg or loss of control of bladder or bowel function secondary to the nerve injury. All other complaints can usually be controlled with conservative measures.

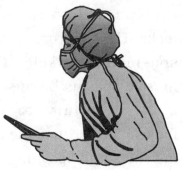

Neck Pain

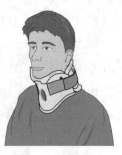

Herniated discs in the neck present with the same type of symptoms. The pain starts in the middle of the neck and radiates down one or both arms. The pain can also radiate up over the top of the head. This is called a cervogenic headache. The step treatments for this pain are the same as the treatments for the lower back. The epidural steroid injection in the neck is slightly more risky than in the lower back. Take care to find a provider that is familiar with the technique.

Back Pain

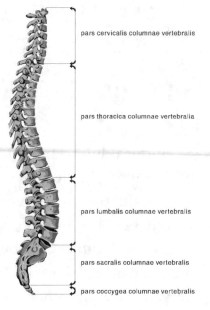

pars cervicalis columnae vertebralis

pars thoracica columnae vertebralia

pars lumbalis columnae vertebralis

pars sacralis columnae vertebralis

pars coccygea columnae vertebralis

Non-radiating back pain is also called axial pain. The pain is a belt-like pain across the back and, sometimes, has a small radiating component into the buttocks. The pain comes from spasmodic muscle. The muscle spasms because of a direct injury to the muscle, or because the nerve that controls the muscle instructs it to spasm.

Primary Muscle Spasm

We have all, at one point or another in our life, had lower back pain from overexerting ourselves. Lifting something that is too heavy or trying an athletic activity without the proper warm-up. The pain comes from spasmodic muscle. In most cases, the spasm resolves and the pain goes away quickly. If the pain does not go away, then the next step is an anti-inflammatory and/or muscle relaxants. If this is ineffective and the muscle spasms continue, then trigger point and, possibly, botox

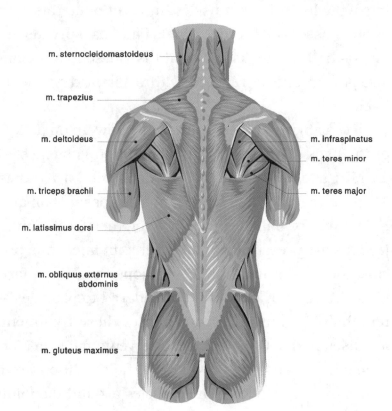

injections can be considered. These options are discussed in detail in Chapter One: Interventional Pain Management.

If there is muscle spasm secondary to the nerves that control the muscle, then the treatment is based on the treatment of the nerve. The most common nerve that causes muscle spasm in the muscles around the spine is the same nerve that also controls the facet joints, that is, the small joints on the side of the spine that help the spine rotate. If the joint has arthritic changes present, the nerve causes the muscles around the spine to spasm. This presents as the same belt-like tightening of the lower back muscles. In addition to this pain, another associated component is pain that spreads into one or both buttocks. The pain is worse if you stand straight up and is relieved with a forward tilt of the back.

The arthritis of these joints will show up on an MRI of the back. Therefore, if this condition is suspected, an MRI should be obtained to determine if it exists. The treatment for this type of muscle spasm is an anti-inflammatory. If ineffective; however, then facet joint injections are prescribed. If the facet joint injections provide adequate relief, but are not long-lived, then facet joint rhizotomies should be considered to provide 4-6 months of continued relief. Both of these treatments are discussed in Chapter One: Interventional Pain Management. Because this is an arthritic condition, exercise is essential to keep the muscles around the joints strong to protect the joints. In general, the stronger the muscles are, the less stress on the joints and, hence, the least amount of degeneration.

Neck Pain

In the neck, the pain is localized to the neck and shoulder area without radiation into the arms or hands. Motion of the neck makes it worse, as does carrying things in your arms. The treatment options for the neck are the same as those for the lower back. Again, due to the proximity to the spine cord, take care to carefully perform these procedures.

Thus, pain in either the neck or lower back, that either does or does not radiate into an extremity, can be treated once the reason for the pain is determined, and the appropriate treatment plan is made.

m. splenius capitis
m. levator scapulae
m. sternocleidomastoideus
m. scalenius anterior
m. scalenus medius
m. scalenus posterior
m. trapezius
m. deltoideus

m. thyrohyoideus
m. omohyoideus
m. sternohyoideus
m. omohyoideus inferior

Notes

Chapter Four

Neurological Approaches to Pain Management (Migraines)

Grace Forde, M.D.

Grace Forde, M.D. is the director of Neurologic services at North American Partners in Pain Management. A graduate of Albert Einstein College of Medicine, she completed her residency in Neurology at the University of California San Diego and her Pain Management and Headache fellowship at the University of California San Francisco. She is a Diplomate of the American Academy of Neurology with subspecialty certification in Pain Management. Dr. Forde is part of a national initiative that trains other physicians in the treatment of chronic pain.

Migraine Headaches

Millions of Americans suffer from headaches, and the most common diagnosis is migraines. It was estimated that 28 million Americans (age 12 and older) suffer from migraines. The breakdown is 21 million females and 7 million males. Migraines are associated with disability and the prevalence peaks in the 25- to 55-age range, which is significant, since the majority of these women have jobs and childcare responsibilities. Migraines are more common than asthma and diabetes combined, yet, less than half of the patients were diagnosed (49%).

One of the reasons migraines remain undiagnosed is that they are often mistaken for other types of headaches such as sinus and tension headaches. Migraines are often mistaken for sinus headaches because the pain can be felt on the face around the eyes and in the sinuses. This occurs because of the relationship of the sinuses and the trigeminal nerve, which is important in the perception of the migraine pain. This type of migraine can include symptoms such as stuffy or runny nose and watery eyes.

Weather changes and "allergies" can be triggers for migraines. Migraines are also mistaken for tension headaches because the pain is felt in the back of the neck and can occur on both sides of the head.

In a recent study, three out of four migraine patients reported neck pain with their migraine attack. Sinus and tension are common triggers for migraines. Other potential triggers for migraines include certain foods and food additives such as caffeine, MSG, nitrites and NutraSweet, bright lights, certain smells and strong odors, skipping meals, loud noises, changes in altitude or barometric pressure, stress, alcohol, changes in sleep habits, and hormonal fluctuations/menstrual cycle.

It is very important for all headache-suffers to keep a detailed headache diary for at least 3 months to determine if there is any particular pattern or triggers for their headaches.

Other myths about migraines that keep both the patient and some doctors from making a diagnosis include:

1)   Myth: All migraines are so severe they require bed rest.

Truth: Migraines can range from mild with no disability to very severe where bed rest is required.

2)   Myth: Migraines always have symptoms like vomiting or aura.

Truth: Only 20% of patients experience an aura.

3)   Myth: I always get my headaches with my period.

Truth: These are menstrual migraines and respond to the acute migraine therapies.

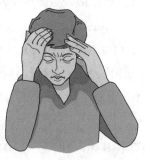

Migraines tend to run in families. If one of your parents suffers from migraines, there is about a 50% higher chance that you will too. A combination of genetic and environmental factors is likely to play a role in the development of migraines.

Cause and Effect

What causes migraines? Most experts believe that migraines are caused by an imbalance of a naturally occurring chemical in the brain called serotonin. This imbalance is believed to cause the blood vessels on the surface of the brain to expand. The expansion of these vessels is what causes the throbbing/pounding headache that many patients with migraines experience. Nerve endings around the blood vessels become inflamed and can lead to the pain and other symptoms associated with migraines.

Migraines are not just headaches. The pain is often, but not always, throbbing or pounding. Patients with migraines have a lower threshold or an increased susceptibility to headaches. Migraine pain can disrupt normal activity and interfere with one's ability to work or enjoy time with family and friends.

Symptoms

Symptoms of migraines include a one-sided headache, which is usually throbbing or pounding, although the pain can be bilateral. Other symptoms include nausea; vomiting; sensitivity to light, sound, and smells;

stuffy and/or runny nose; watery eyes; dizziness; and mood changes.

About one out of five migraine patients experience warning symptoms that last 30 to 60 minutes before the onset of the migraine (aura). These symptoms include flashing lights, bright or dark pulsating spots in front of eyes, tunnel vision (like looking down the barrel of a gun), loss of vision on one side, confusion, lightheadedness, and difficulty concentrating.

In addition, some patients may begin to experience symptoms up to 2 to 3 days before the actual headache pain begins; this is called a prodrome. Some symptoms that are considered a prodrome include increased thirst, increased urination, cravings, and irritability. The typical migraine can last anywhere from 4 hours up to 3 days, and most patients prefer to lie down in a quiet, dark room.

Treatments

Many of the treatments used for migraines affect the blood vessels, the nerves, or certain chemicals such as serotonin. The treatment options for migraines include preventative, abortive, and acute therapies. The preventative medications are used for patients with frequent headaches that are severe and have a long duration. Patients who are experiencing headaches more than 12 days a month or have severe headaches that last a long time and are associated with a lot of disability are started on .

The rational for preventative medication is that it decreases the frequency, severity, and duration of the migraines. Preventative medication also boosts the effect of the acute symptomatic medication. Abortive medications are used in patients who have warning symptom (aura) before the onset of the migraine attack. The acute symptomatic treatment should be taken within 20 to 30 minutes of the onset of the migraine attack to achieve the best results.

When the appropriate acute medications are used, patients can be completely headache free within 30 to 60 minutes. The acute migraine-specific medications consist mainly of the "triptans." These medications also relieve the associated symptoms of migraines such as nausea; vomiting; and sensitivity to light, sound, and smell. The "triptans" include, in order of FDA (food and drug administration) approval, Sumatriptan (Imitrex), Zolmatriptan (Zomig), Naratriptan (Amerge), Rizatriptan (Maxalt), Almotriptan (Axert), Frovatriptan (Frova), and Eletriptan (Relpax). Patients with uncontrolled hypertension and coronary artery disease should not use the "triptans."

Other medications that are extremely useful include those that are used to treat nausea and vomiting. Over-the-counter medications such as the non-steroidal anti-inflammatory drugs (NSAID), which include Ibuprofen, Advil, Aleeve, and Motrin can be helpful in treating a migraine attack because inflammation of the nerves is part of the mechanism of a migraine attack. Aspirin and Tylenol is less effective. Excedrin and Excedrin

Migraine can be effective if used infrequently for mild headaches, but there is a potential for rebound headaches if used more than one to two times per week. The main reason why Excedrin causes more rebound headaches than any of the other over-the-counter medications is because it contains caffeine.

Many patients like the idea of using herbal or "natural" medicines to treat whatever ales them, and lots of anecdotal evidence exists that shows these medicines are effective, but natural methods should be used under the supervision of a health care provider.

Vitamin B6 can be effective for migraines that mainly occur around the time of the menses. The recommended dose is 50 mg. However, some patients believe that since this is a vitamin, more must be better, and end up taking more than the recommended dose, which can cause a peripheral neuropathy (a problem with the nerves in the foot).

Feverfew, a mildly stimulating anti-migraine herb, which is a "naturally occurring" anti-inflammatory substance, has been effective, but was also associated with rebound headaches. In my experience, the herbal medications/vitamins magnesium, coenzyme Q10, folic acid, and riboflavin are helpful in the treatment of migraines.

Rebound headaches are headaches that occur daily because of frequent use of acute symptomatic medications. Excedrin and prescription medications used to treat migraines such as Fioricet, Fiorinal, Esgic, and certain other medications such as anti-hypertensives are associated with a high potential for rebound headaches. To prevent rebound headaches, acute medications should not be used more than two times a week or more than eight times a month, and patients with more frequent headaches should be started on preventative medication.

Warning Signs

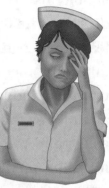

Most migraines are stereotypic, which means the patient usually experiences the same symptoms with each attack. However, different symptoms can occur at different times in the course of the disease. There are particular warning signs that patients need to be aware of that might indicate a more serious condition than a migraine. These signs include blacking out; episodes of confusion; drowsiness; difficulty speaking; changes in personality; and weakness or numbness involving the face, arms, or legs.

If you are over 40 and develop headaches for the first time, you experience the worse headache of your life, you get headaches when you cough, exercise, sneeze, strain having a bowel movement or during other strenuous activities, have sex or bend over. They could be benign exertional headaches, but you may have something more serious. In general, a new onset headache in someone who does not usually get headaches, a headache much more severe than usual, a significant change in a typical headache, or a headache that escalates more rapidly than usual or steadily over days should be evaluated medically as soon as possible.

Patients with migraines should maintain regular sleeping patterns and regular eating patterns. They should also get regular exercise, all of which will help decrease the frequency of the attacks. Patients should learn to recognize their triggers and avoid them. Always take your medication as directed by your health care provider, and keep your migraine medicine with you at all times so that you can take it at the first sign of headache pain. You should expect complete relief from you migraine medication within 2 hours after taking the medication.

Treatment of migraines should include both pharmacologic and non-pharmacologic (non-medication) strategies. Non-pharmacologic techniques include relaxation techniques, guided imagery, biofeedback, cognitive therapy psychotherapy, lifestyle changes, acupuncture, acupressure, physical and massage therapies, trigger point injections, botux, and transcutaneous electrical nerve stimulation (TENS).

The Misdiagnosis of Migraines with Sinus Headache

Sinus problems rarely cause headaches unless the patient has an acute sinus infection. A headache specialist and family practitioner advertised in the newspaper for people with self-diagnosed sinus headaches. Ninety-six of those who responded actually had migraines or probable migraines. Most of the headaches are, indeed, migraines even though most patients and most physicians think they are sinus headaches.

Blockage of the sinus drainage system can cause infection, and these infections are classified as acute sinusitis. Acute sinusitis is generally associated with fever, pain over the sinuses, and a yellow-green bad tasting or smelling discharge from the nose and back of the throat. A headache associated with fever and/or signs of infection must be evaluated and treated immediately.

Ears, nose, and throat physicians do not recognize headache as a major symptom in the diagnosis of sinusitis. They list it as a minor symptom along with bad breath and fatigue. Chronic low-grade inflammation of the sinuses can very rarely cause headaches. However, a severe sinus problem can cause a migraine attack. One of the distinguishing features between migraines and acute sinus headache is the nasal discharge. Patients with acute sinus infection have

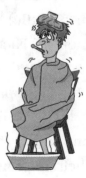

a yellow-greenish nasal discharge, while those with migraines have a clear discharge. Allergies to pollen, grass, and hay fever rarely cause headaches unless patients develop an acute sinus infection.

The Misdiagnosis of Migraines as Tension Headaches

Tension-type headaches are the most common types of headaches. Probably 90% or more of the world's population has experienced one from time-to-time. Many of these headaches are associated with tension in the muscles in the head, face, jaw, or neck, although this may not be the case in some patients. There is much speculation whether tension-type headaches and migraines are separate disorders. Some headache specialists believe they are caused by similar mechanisms, and most patients experience both types of headaches with tension headaches sometimes triggering a migraine.

Tension headaches can be episodic (occurring once in a while) or chronic (occurring most days of the month). Factors that potentially confound the diagnosis of migraines include stress, bilateral or non-throbbing head pain, and the presence of neck pain. Stress is the most frequently reported trigger of migraines. In one study, 75% of the patients reported neck pain with their migraines. Nausea; vomiting; and sensitivity to light, sound, and smell are usually not associated features of a tension-type headache.

Early theories of the causes of tension-type headaches reveal that the pain is due to contraction of the muscles around the head and neck, which might explain why this type of headache was originally called muscle contraction headaches. It is true that people who tighten up the muscles around the head, neck, and shoulders can experience headaches. Other potential triggers for tension-type headaches include poor posture, tightening of the jaw, arthritis of the neck, using the computer for prolonged periods of time, and talking on the telephone with the phone cradled between the ear and shoulder. Many patients develop an acute tension-type headache that, over a period of hours, can develop into a full-blown migraine attack.

Depression and anxiety are often associated with migraines and tension-type headaches and should be addressed as part of the patient's headache picture. Some patients with depression and anxiety will need medication or treatment by a clinical psychologist.

Psychology

Patients with chronic pain, defined as pain that persists for 3 months after healing has occurred, usually experience a lot of depression and anxiety. Patients with chronic pain experience sleep disturbance, decreased libido (sex drive), appetite changes, and an increased focus on minor aches and pain, which is part of every-day living. Patients' emotions, culture, past pain experience, expectations, and environment all play a part in the chronic pain process. For the majority of patients, the pain is usually the first event and the depression and anxiety is secondary. However, patients with a primary diagnosis of anxiety and depression can also experience pain as a secondary phenomenon. It is sometimes unclear whether the pain or the depression or anxiety came first, but it is well established that they all interact to make each condition worse.

Once established, both the pain and the depression or anxiety need to be treated aggressively. A multidisciplinary pain center is a facility where patients are evaluated by a pain management specialist, as well as a pain psychologist or a pain psychiatrist. These specialists determine whether the patient needs ongoing psychological intervention. In addition to treating the anxiety and depression, the psychological evaluation determines whether certain pain behaviors are present, and a treatment strategy is then developed.

Patients usually learn coping skills and participate in cognitive behavioral therapy. One of the main goals of psychological approaches is to teach patients techniques to help them manage their condition appropriately. For example, a specific type of biofeedback training is frequently used and can be especially effective in treating muscle contraction headaches. Cognitive approaches and hypnosis usually focus on feelings of distress and discomfort. Medication management for the psychological component of pain is an integral part, but not the only part of a multidisciplinary pain program.

Acupuncture

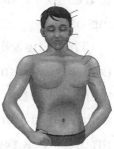

The word acupuncture was introduced by French Jesuits from the Latin acus (needle) and puncture (puncture). The earliest reports noted techniques of diagnosis by feeling the pulse, consuming medicinal herbs and teas, practicing health promotion, and using glass needles. Widespread awareness of acupuncture started in 1971, when it was reported in the New York Times that a patient had his postoperative pain alleviated by three acupuncture needles. Since then, acupuncture has been transformed by the intellects and experiences of western physicians, so that most of the acupuncture practiced here in the United States is a hybrid between traditional Chinese medicine and biomedical science. In 1973, reports indicated that 15 to 25% of all surgery performed in the major hospitals in China were performed by using acupuncture analgesia with a 90% success rate.

Both acupuncture and complimentary medicine can be incorporated successfully into a multidisciplinary pain program. Acupuncture appears to activate the body's own pain relieving substances, called opioids. These opioids are the morphine-like drugs that our bodies produce. Serotonin (important in migraines) and other chemicals are released when acupuncture is used to treat pain. Acupuncture can be very effective in treating pain.

There have been several controlled trials using acupuncture for analgesia in different pain states. These include, but are not limited to, low back pain, headache and craniofacial pain, preoperative pain, osteoarthritis, neck pain, tennis elbow, musculoskeletal pain (such as fibromyalgia), sickle cell anemia crises, post herpetic neuralgia, and complex regional pain syndrome (CRPS).

Other non-painful conditions that can be helped by acupuncture include, asthma, postoperative- and chemotherapy-induced nausea, gynecologic and obstetrics problems such as infertility, painful menses, and postmenopausal symptoms. One study showed that acupuncture can shorten the labor in women who are having their first baby; however, acupuncture can induce abortion if used earlier in pregnancy before labor has begun. Acupuncture can also be effective in patients who have had a stroke, head trauma, urinary tract disorders, chest pain related to heart disease, tinnitus (ringing in the ear), constipation, and/or depression.

Many patients report a feeling of well being or relaxation following an acupuncture treatment, especially if electrical stimulation was used. Some patients report lightheadedness, anxiety, agitation, or tearfulness. The sense of relaxation can sometimes evolve into a feeling of fatigue or depression, which can last for several days.

Contact dermatitis from the needles has also been reported. Minor bruising at the needle sites is not uncommon and extensive hematomas are possible, especially in patients on blood thinners. Soreness of the muscles that have been needled is common during the first days following treatment, and it is possible that the acupuncture treatment can temporarily exacerbate the symptoms that were being treated. Other risks involve fainting, infection, or puncture of an internal organ. Pneumothorax (puncture of the lung) is the most frequently reported and the most easily produced serious complication.

Various types of infection can occur such as hepatitis B, HIV disease, infection of the bone (osteomyelitis), and infection of the lining of the heart (endocarditis). These can be avoided if sterile techniques are observed and needles are not reused. Patients with pacemakers should not receive electrical stimulation across the chest.

Most patients see results in about eight to ten sessions, but if no improvement is seen after the tenth treatment, it is unlikely that you will benefit from this form of intervention. Initially, patients are seen three to four times a week, and then the frequency is decreased as the pain subsides.

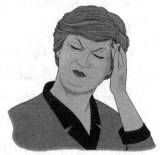

Complimentary Medicine

Complimentary medicine, also referred to as alternative or natural medicine, has been in existence for centuries. Supporting organ structure and function and nutrient status repletion can make the individual more resistant to illness, improve quality of life and, hopefully, reduce or eliminate life limiting symptoms. To look at disease as only a set of symptoms to be blocked by the actions of a certain drug or herb limits our ability to understand the nature of disease. At times, recommendations in complimentary medicine are intended to strengthen health and vitality.

Natural therapeutics can be used as a first line of defense for common complaints and conditions where people use over-the-counter medications (OTC), for people who prefer a natural agent, or individuals in whom OTC is contraindicated; e.g., an arthritis patient with a kidney disorder should avoid the typical OTC medications except for Tylenol and might benefit from a trial of glocosamine and chondroitin. A pilot with a cold could benefit from Echinacea and vitamin C, thus avoiding the sedating effects of antihistamine and decongestants.

Natural therapeutics can be used to compliment traditional medical care. For example, ginkgo biloba, avmil, and cordyceps sinesis can be used to counter the decrease in sexual libido that can possibly occur when using some of the medications commonly prescribed to treat chronic pain. Another example is the use of milk thistle to protect the liver when patients are taking drugs that elevate liver enzymes and stress liver detoxification pathways such as Tylenol-containing products.

Vitamin E, used as an anti-aging agent, and calcium and magnesium, used to prevent osteoporosis, are examples of natural agents used in preventative ways to promote health and well being. Certain medications can deplete nutrients; for example, oral contraceptives can deplete magnesium, folic acid, and vitamin B6 and B12. Interestingly, these are the main vitamin supplements prescribed for patients with menstrual migraines.

The World Health Organization defines herbal supplementation as: Finished labeled medicinal products that contain, as active ingredients, aerial or underground parts of plants, or other plant material, or combination thereof, whether crude state or as plant preparation. Plant material includes juices, gums, fatty oils, essential oils, and any other substances of this nature. Herbal supplements may contain excipients, in addition to the active ingredients. Medicine-containing plant material combined with chemically defined substances including chemically defined, isolated constituents of plants are not considered to be herbal supplements. Exceptionally, in some countries, herbal supplements may also contain, by tradition, natural organic or inorganic active ingredients, which are not of plant origin.

Examples of plant-derived medications include:
- Aspirin was derived from the white willow bark

- Caffeine was derived from coffee shrub
- Colchicine was derived from autumn crocus
- Cromolyn was derived from khella
- Cyclosporine was derived from cordyceps
- Digoxin was derived from foxglove
- Morphine was derived from opium poppy
- Quinine was derived from cinchona bark
- Taxol was derived from pacific yew
- Theophylline was derived from tea shrub
- Vincristine was derived from periwinkle

Herbs are natural products, but the composition is not standardized. The constituents can vary depending on genetic factors, climate and soil where the plants are grown, and various other external factors. As a result, herbal supplements, when processed, can contain harmful agents or very little of the herb itself. Therefore, herbs can be ineffective for this reason or can, in fact, be harmful because of the adulterants. Some tips for buying herbs include:

- Find a retailer whose product selection meets you needs and whose staff is knowledgeable
- Find a physician or other healthcare professional that is knowledgeable about herbs to avoid potentially dangerous side effects and interactions.
- Ask your pharmacist or other healthcare provider for product information, recommended doses, interactions, side effects and effectiveness
- Do not use supplements during pregnancy and while you are breast feeding except with the advice of a physician

- Individuals with serious health conditions should not use herbal supplements except with the advice and supervision of a qualified healthcare provider
- Be aware that there are sub-therapeutic products on the shelf and misleading the consumer is a common occurrence.

Use general caution when using herbs; for example, use with extreme caution in children younger than 2 years of age, and note that large and prolonged doses of herbs increase the potential for adverse events. Remember, more isn't always better. Vitamin B6 in the recommended dose of 50 mg is usually well tolerated and safe, but in higher doses can cause numbness and tingling of the feet, a form of peripheral neuropathy. Excess licorice can lower the potassium levels, and ginkgo biloba can cause bleeding if taken with medications such as aspirin, ibuprofen, or Coumadin.

There are specific recommendations for different disease processes, but that is beyond the scope of this chapter.

Notes

Chapter Five
Medications for Pain Management

Mary Milano Carter, APRN, BC, MS

Mary Milano Carter, APRN, BC, MS is the Nurse Practitioner and Director of Clinical Services for North American Partners in Pain Management. She completed her Master of Science and Nurse Practitioner degrees at Adelphi University in Garden City, NY and has been a Registered Nurse for 17 years. She is Board Certified as an Adult Nurse Practitioner, Gerontological Nurse, and Medical-Surgical Nurse. She is the founding President of the American Society for Pain Management Nursing–Long Island Chapter and has been an active member of the American Society for Pain Management Nursing, the Oncology Nursing Society, The New York State Nurse Practitioner Association, and Sigma Theta Tau International Honor Society for Nursing for many years.

Medications for Pain

Many options are available to help control chronic pain without the use of medications. Some sufferers may need to take medication for a short time. Others, however, who have failed other means at controlling or reducing pain, may be candidates for chronic medication therapy. This scares some patients, as most people relate narcotics to pain. It is true that narcotics are used to treat pain, but many other effective medications are also available!

Common concerns from patients include being labeled a drug seeker or complainer if they ask for pain medications. In reality, if a patient is in pain and seeks medical attention for pain, he or she has the right to ask for medication. Some patients fear they will lose control of themselves while taking medications. Remember, the point of taking an extensive history and physical on a patient is not only to properly diagnose the pain, but also to determine treatment as well.

With medications, providers start with the basics and add, delete, and bring medication doses up and down very slowly. This process is used to assess what is working and not working, as well as to identify and manage side effects and allergic reactions. Other patients' express that they are anxious about pain not responding to medication. This is another reason for the start low–go slow approach that providers take with medication management.

Why take a pill on a daily basis if it is not working? Medical management of pain is not "cookie cutter." It is trial and error, until the doctors find a medication or combination of medications that work. The most frightening thing to patients is being labeled a drug addict or literally becoming addicted to medications. In point of fact, multiple studies have confirmed that many patients have valid reasons to take opiates and other medications for pain. When taken properly, as prescribed, outcomes have shown that less than 1% of the people who take these medications actually become addicts.

The World Health Organization (WHO) has a step approach to pain management. It is called the WHO Analgesic Ladder and was created to help patients suffering from cancer pain. It is now also used as a template for treating non-cancer pain. The first step is treating pain when it is mild. Medications here include non-narcotic options such as acetaminophen and non-steroidal anti-inflammatory drugs (NSAIDs). Sometimes, adjuvant (additional non-narcotic) medications are added at this level. If pain persists, a narcotic or "opioid" is given in addition to the existing medications. Usually, this is a short acting medication, designed to last only 2 to 3 hours in the body. If this is not successful, the patient progresses to step three, which is the addition of stronger opioid medications, usually in the long acting form.

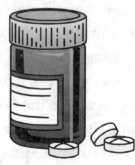

The First Step

Basic medications taken for pain consist of acetaminophen (Tylenol), aspirin, salicylates, and NSAIDs. Many are over-the-counter, which means they are available without a prescription. Many still come in prescription strength. These medications are first line for complaints of pain, usually started with the over-the-counter variety by the patient. They can be changed to stronger, more effective prescription NSAIDs by the provider and be given in conjunction with other medications (adjuvants). There is no risk of physical or psychological dependence with these medications. They can be started and stopped at any time. There is, what is known as, a "ceiling effect" with these medications, which means that taking three or more pills will not make patients feel any better than the suggested one or two.

Acetaminophen is a wonderful painkiller and fever reducer; however, it does not have any anti-inflammatory properties. Studies have determined that the maximum daily dose of acetaminophen for an adult is 4,000 mg. If patients are taking two, 500 mg tablets of acetaminophen every six hours on a daily basis, they are reaching the maximum dose. If they also take other pills that contain acetaminophen, like many over-the-counter preparations, they are exceeding the daily dose. This puts patients at risk for kidney and liver dysfunction.

Other factors such as daily alcohol intake and other existing medical conditions such as high blood pressure, diabetes, and hepatitis can also compound this risk. The Food and Drug Administration (FDA) estimates that taking acetaminophen with three or more alcoholic beverages daily can greatly increase the risk of liver damage. Furthermore, kidney function normally decreases every year with age. Maximum daily acetaminophen intake should be lowered to 2,000 to 3,000 mg per day in the elderly for safety's sake.

Aspirin (Bayer) is also a wonderful painkiller and fever reducer. The maximum daily dose, like acetaminophen, is 4,000 mg. Aspirin has a side effect; however, it decreases the way that platelets clump together in the bloodstream. Platelets play an important role in the way blood clots. This effect on platelets is why many patients are placed on an aspirin a day to thin the blood for the positive heart and vascular effects. The negative side effect is that bleeding time is longer than usual. Aspirin can also effect the stomach and may cause bleeding or an ulcer. Aspirin tablets are available; however, with an enteric coating; that is, an outside layer on the tablet to protect the stomach lining.

Salicylates are painkillers similar to aspirin. Prescription salicylates such as diflunisal (Dolobid) and choline magnesium (Trilisate) are old and proven medications. There is a reduced risk of stomach effect and no effect, whatsoever, on platelets in the bloodstream. Non-steroidal anti-inflammatory medications (NSAIDS) are popular painkillers, with MANY prescription NSAIDs distributed over-the-counter in the past decade. The misinformed public, unfortunately, over utilizes these medications to the point that risk of stomach problems and bleeding outweighs the benefit of pain relief. It is estimated that 103,000 patients are hospitalized each year in the United States with NSAID-related gastrointestinal issues, with treatment costing upwards of 2 billion dollars. This has resulted in approximately 16,500 deaths per year.

Of the older NSAIDs, ibuprofen has proved to be the safest, with the lowest risk of bleeding, among all the NSAIDs available. If patients are taking any prescription or even over-the-counter NSAIDs on a routine basis for greater than six weeks, they should also be taking an additional medication to protect their stomach. Many of these are also available over-the-counter. Patients should consider a stomach protecting medication if they take a daily steroid pill, have a history of stomach or intestinal bleeding, or are elderly. It is not advised to remain on a daily NSAID for greater than three months, no matter what the age or medical history.

Popular over-the-counter NSAIDs include ibuprofen (Motrin, Advil), which should not exceed 200 mg to 400 mg every four hours as needed; naproxen sodium (Alleve, Naprosen) dosed at 250 mg every six hours as needed, and ketoprophen (Orudis), which can be taken at 35 to 50 mg every six hours as needed. These medications also come in prescription strength higher doses, but should only be taken under the direction of a provider. There are other prescription, more potent NSAIDs such as indomethacin (Indocin), diclofenac (Voltaren,

Cataflam), etodolac (Lodine), meloxicam (Mobic), and ketorolac (Toradol) that can only be taken for a short period of time. Currently, ketorolac is the only intravenous NSAID that is widely used in hospitals for postoperative pain.

A newer generation of NSAIDs is available, by prescription only, better known as COX 2 inhibitors. COX stands for cyclooxygenase, which is an isoenzyme in the body. The traditional NSAIDs previously mentioned are COX 1 inhibitors. COX 1 and 2 are responsible for a chemical reaction at the cell level in the body that produces a chemical called "prostaglandins." Prostaglandins have a vital function; that is, they are responsible for the upkeep of certain tissues in the body. The unfortunate side effect of prostaglandins is their effect on sensory nerves. Prostaglandins make sensory nerves more aware of painful impulses.

COX 1 maintains the stomach lining. When this isoenzyme is affected by the COX 1 NSAID to avoid the effect on the sensory nerves, the protection of the stomach lining is altered as well. This is why many patients who take NSAIDs frequently have stomachaches and potential ulcers. When the COX 2 isoenzyme is interrupted from the nerve pain, it does not protect the stomach; therefore, a reduced risk of having any stomach side effects exists. These newer COX 2 inhibitors include celecoxib (Celebrex), rofecoxib (Vioxx), and valdecoxib (Bextra). These are effective without the typical side effects. A pharmaceutical company is currently working on an intravenous form of the COX 2 NSAIDs that will certainly be used in the hospital setting. Rofecoxib was recently pulled off the market by the manufacturer due to increased risk of heart attack. There is still a lot of uncertainty about COX 2 inhibitors and those drugs increasing the risk of stroke and heart attack. Seek the advice of your doctor before considering this type of treatment.

The Second Step

If the first step is not effective, or not very effective, stronger medications can be started or added to the mix. Tramadol is a newer pain medication that comes in a preparation with and without acetaminophen. The daily limit is 4,000 mg, but only 3,000 in the elderly. This is because tramadol can potentially lower the seizure threshold. In other words, a slight chance of having a seizure exists, even if the patient has never had one before. Also, taking certain popular prescription antidepressants along with tramadol can lower the seizure threshold and should NEVER be prescribed together.

Tramadol is a short-acting medication, which means that it should be taken as needed for pain. It helps ease the pain, but should be out of the patient's system in a few hours. The same is true for short-acting narcotics or opiates. The main reason to turn to opiates is non-opiate medication failure. A short-acting opiate may be started, and the patient's progress watched closely. Like tramadol, most short-acting opiate medications are mixed with acetaminophen, and some are even mixed with aspirin or ibuprofen. This mixture limits the number of pills a patient can take a day.

These medications should be taken as needed, starting at a low dose, and titrate upwards (taking more) as needed. It is particularly important, at this time, that providers know what other medications the patient has taken in the past to help with drug selection and dose. Opiates have side effects including sedation, constipation, nausea, edema of the extremities (swelling), respiratory depression (slowed breathing), urine retention, pruritis (itch), and hyper excitability (jumpy feeling).

All side effects should subside, with time, as the patient continues to take the medication, except for constipation. Remember, constipation is like pain, it is easier to prevent than to treat! Constipation should first be managed with a change in diet to include high fiber and fluid intake. If this fails, over-the-counter fiber supplements and stool softeners can be added. Laxatives should be avoided unless necessary. Prescription constipation medications are also available.

Other medications can be added to the drug regimen to treat other side effects as well. But why treat the side effects and not take the patient off of the opiate? If the patient is getting adequate relief of pain from the opiate medication, it is worth adding another medication to control the side effect. Effective medications are available to counter react and/or decrease sedation, edema, nausea, pruritis, and hyper excitability. It is important to note that side effects from medications are different from allergic reactions. True allergies produce symptoms such as a red raised rash or throat swelling to the point of having difficulty breathing.

So how do opiates work in the body? In the back of the spinal cord, the peripheral (coming in from the body) nerves meet the central nervous system nerves. At this synapse, or space, a chemical called substance P is released. Substance P is the chemical that helps transmit (pass on) pain signals up to the brain. Opiates bind to receptors at the space where substance P is released, thereby, inhibiting the substance P.

Short acting opiates include propoxyphene, oxycodone, hydrocodone, codeine, hydromorphone, meperidine, fentanyl, and morphine. Propoxyphene comes in a mixed tablet with acetaminophen (Darvocet N100 or Darvocet A500) or aspirin (Darvon N). It is not a particularly effective painkiller. If taken for an extended period of time, the breakdown of propoxyphene, norpropoxyphene in the body can build up in the bloodstream and cause problems such as convulsions.

Hydrocodone is more potent that propoxyphene and comes in mixed tablets with acetaminophen (Vicodin, Norco, Lorcet, Lortab, Maxidone, Zydone) and ibuprofen (Vicoprofen). Hydrocodone is not marketed without acetaminophen or ibuprofen. The most popular hydrocodone tablets are Vicodin, which comes in multiple strengths. Unfortunately, there is a large amount of acetaminophen in all Vicodin strengths.

Codeine is marketed alone and mixed with acetaminophen (Tylenol #3 and #4). It is the most constipating and nauseating of the opiates. It is the only member of this drug class that has a maximum daily dose (120 mg) because of the side effects. Codeine is also popular in prescription cough syrups becasue it is a wonderful cough suppressant. What most people do not know about codeine is that the liver's enzyme system, which breaks down all medications in the body, converts codeine to morphine in the body. Approximately 10 % of the Caucasian population lacks the enzyme responsible for this conversion. In this case, the codeine would not produce any pain relief. Also, if the person taking codeine has a true allergy to morphine, he or she may also react to the codeine.

Meperidine (Demerol) is better known for it's injectable form, which is sometimes used for acute postoperative pain. It is also available in tablet form. Meperidine is not very potent and is rarely used in chronic pain management. The use of meperidine, in general, has become controversial. Recent studies have shown that prolonged use can cause a build up of the breakdown of meperidine, normeperidine in the bloodstream. Normeperidine, in high amounts, can cause seizures and possible death. Most hospitals only allow doses of meperidine for surgical pain; however, only for 48 hours or less, the timeframe deemed safe through studies.

The Third Step

Medications in the third step are extremely potent narcotics and are only uses for patients who are opiate tolerant; that is, the patient is accustomed to taking opiates. In this step, determining medication should be based on previous narcotic use. It is time to change opiates if the patient is taking the maximum daily dose of a medication from step two. Taking the medication on a steady basis everyday, and the amount of acetaminophen intake per day is also an indicator to move up.

It is important to note here that if you are taking an opiate on a steady basis, do not stop taking it abruptly. You risk experiencing symptoms of narcotic withdrawal such as anxiety, headache, chills, joint and muscle pains, runny nose, nausea, vomiting, abdominal cramping, and diarhhea. Opiate medications should always be tapered back slowly over time, just as they were tapered up slowly over time.

Hydromorphone (Dilaudid) is a straight narcotic tablet and is five times more potent than morphine, milligram for milligram. This medication is used for patients who have already been on steady doses of narcotics. It comes in a short-acting form, which lasts about two hours in the body. The long-acting form, Palladone, which is a 24-hour capsule, was just approved for sale by the FDA.

Oxycodone comes alone in tablet, capsule, and elixer forms, mixed with aspirin (Percodan) or acetaminophen (Percocet and others). A long-acting form of oxycodone is also available (also known as OxyContin). This medication is designed to slowly

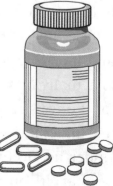

release oxycodone in the body over a 12-hour period, to prevent pain instead of treating the pain. Medications such as this, with a sustained release mechanism, should never be crushed, chewed, or split in half. In doing so, the sustained release mechanism is broken, and the patient risks getting a large dose of medication very rapidly. This can have serious effects such as respiratory depression and death. Patients who are taking large doses of short-acting pain medications, on a daily basis, are switched over to long-acting medications for better pain relief and ease of taking the medication.

Morphine also comes in long- and short-acting formulations. Morphine has always been the "gold standard" in pain medications to which all other narcotics are compared. All short-acting morphines are acetaminophen free and include capsules (MSIR) and an elixer (Roxanol). A few long-acting morphines are available including MS Contin, Oramorph, and Kadian, which release morphine over 8 to 12 hours, and a newer formulation called Avinza, which is a 24-hour capsule is available as well. Morphine also has an active metabolite called 6 morphine glucoranide, which can build up in the bloodstream.

Fentanyl is another pain medication with a short- and long-acting preparation. The long-acting formula is actually in a patch form that is worn by the patient for 3 days straight (Duragesic). The fentanyl is deposited under the skin and is picked up by the bloodstream. Under no circumstances should opiate-naïve patients be started on a fentanyl patch. Patients MUST be taking 60 mg of morphine, or the equivalent in another mediation, to start on the lowest dose of this patch. The oral form is an oral unit (similar to a lollipop). This gained FDA approval only for cancer pain. This potent unit is absorbed through the membranes on the inside of the mouth directly into the bloodstream. Studies have shown that this medication is as fast acting as the intravenous morphine given in hospitals. It is raspberry flavored and very sweet because of the two grams of sugar used to make each unit. Patients using this medication need to have good oral care, brushing teeth and rinsing frequently because studies have shown an increase in cavities with the use of this medication.

Last, but not least, methadone is another long-acting pain medication. Many patients cringe when methadone (Dolophine) is mentioned because it is frequently used for addicts who are withdrawing from heroine. In reality, methadone was created as a pain medication during World War II. It is a highly effective painkiller with less sedation side effects than the others. Methadone can, however, cause cardiac side effects in higher doses, and anyone taking this medication should be monitored appropriately. One last thing to mention about long-acting narcotics is the fact that no patient should ever take these for acute pain.

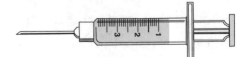

Opiate Medications NOT for Use in Chronic Pain Management

A class of narcotic painkillers called mixed opiates is also available. These are not for use in chronic pain patients. They are a mixture of an opiate agonist (narcotic medication) and an opiate antagonist (medication that reverses the effect of narcotics). These medications work well for very short-term acute pain, for example, labor and delivery in the hospital. Anesthesiologists also use them, sometimes, for patients waking up from anesthesia. If a chronic pain patient who has been maintained on opiates takes one of these medications, the patient risks being thrown into withdrawal and severe pain returning from the action of the opiate antagonist. These medications include nalbuphine (Nubain), pentazocine (Talwin NX), and butorphanol (Stadol).

Adjuvant Medications

Many adjuvant medications for pain management exist. These are non-narcotic and are added, deleted, and titrated up and down at all three steps of the WHO ladder. Some have gained FDA approval for use in pain management, and some are used "off label." This means that the medication has been proven effective against pain over years of use in patients, but does not carry an FDA approval for pain. If patients are placed on an off-label medication, providers should discuss this with them. Adjuvant medications come from many different drug categories. These include anticonvulsants, transdermals, steroids, muscle relaxants, triptans, beta-blockers, and botulinum toxin.

Anticonvulsants are medications to control seizures. The ones that are FDA approved for pain are gabapentin (Neurontin), carbamezapine (Tegretol), divalproex (Depakote), and dibenzazapine (Carbatrol). These medications are exceptionally effective against nerve pain (burning, shooting, or dull aching). They should be taken on a daily basis and worked up to an effective dose. Side effects include headache, transient dizziness, hair loss, and bleeding gums at the higher doses.

Transdermals are medications that are absorbed through the skin from a patch or cream form. A popular patch now available is made of 5% lidocaine (Lidoderm), and an effective cream is also available that contains lidocaine and prilocaine (Emla). Lidocaine and prilocaine are both local anesthetics; similar to the novacaine received at the dentist. These medications work for pain locally and have very little to no systemic absorption (going into the rest of the body). Therefore, few side effects occur from these medications.

Another excellent cream product for pain is capsaicin (Zostrix, Tiger Balm), which is available over-the-counter. Capsaicin is actually crushed hot chili peppers and is especially effective for arthritic pains when applied to joints. It comes in oil-based formulations, which means the capsaicin will not wash off the hands with soap and water. Patients need a solvent remover such as turpentine. This is important to mention because any contact with mucous membranes from the fingers that applied the capsaicin will really burn. This includes eyes, nasal passages, inside of the mouth, and genitals. Transdermals must also be applied to intact skin to work effectively.

Steroids are wonderful for short-term use of treating pain from an inflammatory condition such as arthritis. With both short- and long-term use of steroids, side effects are always a possible risk. Short-term use side effects are hormonally charged, usually affecting females, and can cause an irregular menstrual cycle, bloating, water weight gain, mood swings, increased appetite, facial hair, and insomnia (difficulty sleeping). Sounds a little like premenstrual syndrome?

If the patient is a diabetic, short-term steroid use may also increase blood sugars temporarily, with the return to normal soon after taken off the medication. Long-term steroid use brings the potential for much more serious side effects, affecting both males and females. These include weight gain, bone loss and possible osteoporosis, diabetes, high blood pressure, skin problems, stomach ulcers, and a suppressed immune system leaving the patient at risk for infections. These medications include dexamethasone (Decadron), deltasone (Prednisone) and methylprednisolone (Solumedrol).

Muscle relaxants are typically used as adjuvants in treating pain from muscles such as fibrolyalgia syndrome. These medications relax muscles and ease pain and soreness. The biggest side effect from muscle relaxants is sleepiness, so most patients cannot tolerate them during the day. Taken at bedtime, they can help muscle pain, as well as help sleep. Muscle relaxants are available by prescription only and range from very old to very new tablets. Some of the older relaxers include cyclobenzaprine (Flexeril), methocarbamol (Robaxin), and lioresal (Baclofen). The newer relaxers include orphenadrine (Norflex), metalaxone (Skelaxin), and tizanadine (Zanaflex). Metalaxone is not as sedating as the others, and many patients can tolerate this during the day.

Another muscle relaxant called carisoprodol (Soma) has been found to be metabolized by the liver to a drug called meprobamate. Meprobamate is not in the muscle relaxant class, but is a benzodiazepine. Benzodiazepines such as diazepam (Valium) and lorazepam (Ativan) are highly addictive and should only be used sparingly. Patients should not remain on muscle relaxants for more than 3 months straight.

Triptans are the newer medications on the market, and they are specifically for end migraine headache pain. These medications work on the vascular system in the body to stop the pain. Patients with high blood pressure or any cardiac disease should not take these medications. Triptans include naratriptan (Amerge), almotriptan (Axert), frovatriptan (Frova), sumatriptan (Imitrex), rizatriptan (Maxalt), and zolmitriptan (Zomig). Triptans are taken with the onset of the migraine and can be repeated once in 24 hours. Side effects include fatigue, dry mouth, nausea, and chest tightness.

Beta-blockers are actually cardiac medications that have gained approval for the prevention of migraine headaches. These medications include timolol (Blocadren) and propanolol (Inderal). Beta blockers are taken on a daily basis. Side effects include low blood pressure and slow heart beat. Botulinum toxin (Botox) injections are also used in pain management for treatment of severe muscle spasm pain. The toxin paralyzes and releases the muscle to ease pain. This effect lasts for approximately 3 to 6 months.

Off-Label Adjuvants

As previously mentioned, medications used for the treatment of pain that carry no indication for the treatment of pain are available. This occurs frequently and should be disclosed to the patient. Tricyclic antidepressants, which are an old class of medications for the treatment of depression, are widely used for nerve pain. These include amatriptyline (Elavil), nortriptyline (Pamelor), desipramine (Norpramin), and sinequan (Doxepin). The most common side effect is sedation, and these medications are, therefore, taken at bedtime to help the patient sleep. Other side effects include dry mouth and low blood pressure.

Another class of antidepressants called selective serotonin reuptake inhibitors (SSRI) has shown some pain-reducing properties as well. Patients taking sertraline (Zoloft) for depression have noticed a decrease in pain. Unfortunately, pain and depression often occur together. Side effects of SSRIs include decreased sex drive, weight gain, and sleepiness.

Some heart medications are also used for pain. Clonidine (Catapres) is a medication typically used for high blood pressure. In its patch form, it can decrease aches and pains, as well as ease symptoms of narcotic withdrawal when a patient is coming off of opiates. Mexiletine (Mexitil) is a medication for heart arrhythmias (irregular heart beat). It is basically lidocaine in the oral form and is used in patients with burning small nerve fiber pain such as diabetic polyneuropathy. With these two medications, the patient's cardiac history is critical as their use may be limited or contraindicated.

Other anticonvulsants are also used to treat pain off label. Medications such as lamotrigine (Lamictal), topiramate (Topamax), oxcarbazepine (Trileptal), zonisamide (Zonegran), and levetiracetam (Keppra) are used for nerve pain. Side effects include dizziness, upset stomach, memory difficulties, agitation, and weight loss. The weight loss side effect has been so impressive that a few of these medications are now used in clinical trials for obese patients.

Things Providers Should Ask

Most patients who take chronic medications for pain are under the care of a provider that specializes in pain management. Patients should not be surprised if providers ask for a signed medication contract. This contract outlines the rules for receiving pain medications on a regular basis. Patients should only be receiving pain medications through one office, for safety's sake; and they must be responsible for maintaining an accurate count of their medications, storing them in a safe place, and keeping scheduled office visits. Most providers will not write prescriptions for pain medication without a face-to-face office evaluation. In addition, most providers will not call in prescriptions to the pharmacy or mail prescriptions. Laws governing controlled substances such as opiates vary from state to state, and providers must comply with them. This helps prevent, as well as identify, abuse.

Physicians and/or nurses may also require a urine sample from patients on pain medication, every so often, to check for opiates. This ensures that the patient is, indeed, using the prescribed pain medications and will prevent, as well as identify, diversion (selling drugs illegally). Physicians may also, periodically, run blood tests to check liver and kidney function, as some of these medications can affect both.

In Summary

Many medications can be used alone or in combination for short- or long-term use to help control pain. Patients should not be afraid to discuss their options with their provider. It is imperative that patients keep an accurate record of what has worked and not worked, as well as side effects and any allergic reactions experienced. It may take some time to find the right combination of medications, but it will happen. And when it does, relief feels so good! Just think of this as "better living through chemistry."

Notes

Chapter Six

Physical Therapy & Rehabilitation in Chronic Pain

Samuel P. Thampi, M.D.

Samuel P. Thampi, M.D. is an Interventional Pain Specialist at Franklin Hospital Medical Ctr, Valley Stream, N.Y. He completed his residency in Physical Medicine and Rehabiliation at St.Vincent's Hospital Medical Ctr, N.Y., and Pain Management fellowship at Emory University, Atlanta, G.A. He is a diplomate of American Board of Physical Medicine and Rehabilitation with added qualification in Pain Mangement. He is a member of North American Spine Society and International Association for Study of Pain.

Physical Therapy & Rehabilitation in Chronic Pain

Physical therapy is one of the oldest and, yet, popular approaches for management of chronic pain and the associated deconditioning. The earliest account of physical therapy dates back to 3000 B.C. when massage treatment, a type of physical therapy, was developed in Egypt to relieve the aches and pains of the Pharaohs.

Subsequently, multiple methods for physical therapy evolved over the decades, and physical therapy now stands as a strong component in the multidisciplinary approach for the management of chronic pain. Physical therapy works in conjunction with complementary methods such as medications and injections for pain control. Physical therapy includes physical modalities, electric stimulation, traction, braces, and exercise. Physical therapy exercises; however, should be used after the pain is controlled to strengthen the injured area.

Physical Modalities

Physical modalities are physical agents, which are externally applied to the painful area to treat areas of pain. The duration of each session for a modality range from 20 to 30 minutes except for one type of modality called ultrasound, which is typically 5 to 10 minutes per session. The modalities include heat, cryotherapy, iontophoresis, and phonophoresis.

Heat

A common question: patients ask me if they should apply heat or cold for their painful condition. The answer depends on the type of problem. Heat is more useful in chronic pain syndromes, while acute inflammatory conditions respond well to cold therapy.

Heat causes increased blood flow to the region and results in the blood washing away the metabolic debris and brings in new tissue-healing substances. Heat decreases the speed of conduction of a type of nerve fiber called Group IIB muscle spindle, which can perpetuate pain through spasms. Heat increases the stretching capabilities of the ligaments, hence the joint can move freely with the application of heat. Heat can also release endorphins, which are a naturally occurring substance in the body that can relieve pain. The optimum temperature in the tissue for therapeutic effect ranges from 40 to 45 degrees Celsius (104-113 degrees Fahrenheit).

Heat as a modality is used in chronic arthritis, tendonitis, bursitis, chronic neck and back pain, and post herpetic neuralgia. Heat has to be used with caution in acute inflammation, peripheral vascular disease, bleeding diathesis, and malignancies because worsening of the condition with heat application can occur. Heat should also be used with caution in patients with impaired sensation and cognitive dysfunctions since there is a risk of heat-induced skin-burn injury. A variety of techniques are available for heat application; these include hot packs, heating pads, paraffin baths, heat lamps, fluidotherapy, and whirlpool baths.

Hot Packs

Hot packs are canvas packs that contain silicon dioxide. They are immersed in hot water tanks that are heated to a temperature of 74.5 degrees Fahrenheit (23.6 degrees Celsius). The hot packs are removed with tongs and covered with several layers of towels and then applied over the painful region. These packs are typically applied under the supervision of a physical therapist. Patients should not lie down on the heat packs because the water can seep into the towels and result in burn injuries to the skin.

Heating Pads

Heating pads can either be an electrically heated pad or hot water circulated heating pads. Electric heating pads are available in most drugstores. Electric heating pads should be used with caution when using moist towels. Patients must ensure that insulation is intact because of the potential risk of electric burns with electric

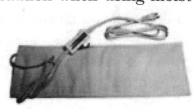

heating pads. Also, do not lie down on the heating pads; risk of localized increase of skin temperature, especially on bony prominences leading to thermal burns, can occur.

Infrared Lamps

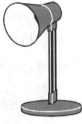

Infrared lamps are lamps with special bulbs that, instead of emitting visible light, emit infra red light that contains a heating property. The infrared lamps are directed toward the

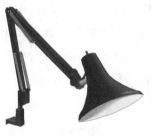

painful joints such as the elbows or hands. Infra red lamps are used on patients who need heat application to the area, cannot tolerate the weight of hot packs, and do not like the idea of hot packs.

Fluidotherapy

For this modality, a special device called a fluidotherapy unit is used. This unit is a special box that contains finely-divided particles that are heated with hot air and constantly circulate in the box from a blast of hot air. On one side of the box, there is an opening to insert the hand or foot that is air proof to the exterior by a fabric attached to the rim that's similar to a glove or boot. The limb is inserted into the box and the heated particles warm the joints (as a result of the heat) and massage the joints as the particles circulate under a blast of heated air.

Paraffin Baths

In this method, paraffin wax is heated in a heating device. The molten wax is applied to the affected area of the body by any of the following three methods: dipping, immersion, and/or brushing. In dipping, the affected area is dipped in the molten wax 7 to 12 times and then covered with plastic or towels to retain the heat. In the immersion technique, the affected area of the body is dipped in the molten wax several times to produce a thin film of wax on the affected area and then immersed in the molten wax for 30 minutes.

The brushing method involves using a paintbrush to apply the molten wax onto the affected area several times and then covered with an insulating material to retain the heat. Typically, the brushing method is preferred in children because they perceive the procedure as fun.

Paraffin wax units are available for use at home. These portable units are heated by electric current to melt paraffin wax. They can be used in the mornings to relieve hand stiffness secondary to osteoarthritis and rheumatoid arthritis. For patients who dislike the smell of traditional paraffin wax, special scented waxes in different fragrances are available to provide a soothing aroma.

Ultrasound

Ultrasound machines use acoustic signals at high frequency (more than 20,000 Hertz). Ultrasound signals generate heat as they pass through the tissues. Ultrasound is a deep-heating modality, compared to the methods described above, and is useful in patients when adipose tissue limits the penetration of heat into the desired joints such as the shoulder, hips, and spine. The duration of application for ultrasound ranges from 5 to 10 minutes, in contrast to other modalities such as heating pads, which are applied for 30 minutes.

Ultrasound should be used with caution in patients with pacemakers, spinal laminectomies with spinal hardware, and/or any internal metallic prostheses or hardware because of the potential risk of overheating the metal-soft tissue junction. Patients with localized cancers to the hip, for example, are at risk using this method because localized heating and increased blood flow to the region can augment the cancer-spread to other unaffected areas.

Sites containing bone cement such as kyphoplasty and vertebroplasty and cemented hip and knee replacements should be avoided because of the possible risk of over heating at the bone-cement junction. Ultrasound for heating is not indicated in children because the ends of the bones (the site of growth or growth plates) can be damaged as a result of local heating and will the stunt the growth of limbs.

Short Wave Diathermy

This method uses deep heating by converting the electric energy to heat energy. The affected area of the body such as the elbow or hand is placed between two plates, and heat is generated by oscillation of an electric field between the plates. Short wave diathermy is used in a wide variety of painful conditions. The typical session ranges between 20 to 30 minutes. All jewelry should be removed during the treatment session because metal on the body can increase the risk of heating. This applies to internal hardware from prior surgeries. Patients with pacemakers should refrain from using this device if the wires or the connection is in the field of the short wave because overheating the wires of the pacemaker can lead to damage of the device.

Cryotherapy (therapeutic use of cold)

Cryotherapy is used in acute musculoskeletal conditions such as sprains and strains, bursitis, tendonitis, acute arthritis, and post-operative spine and joint pain. Cold temperatures decrease the transmission of nerve fibers, which can transmit pain and decrease the function of nerve fibers responsible for spasticity, since muscle spasms can augment and maintain a painful state.

Cold should be used with caution in patients with peripheral vascular disease (PVD); areas with impaired sensation, for example, a numb leg or hand as a result of nerve damage; and/or patients with cognitive impairment or communication disorders, as they are prone to frostbite. Patients with Cryoglobulinemia, Raynaud's disease, and cold induced urticaria are at risk for exacerbating their symptoms.

Cool Packs

Cool packs include commercially available, chemi-cal gel packs, which contain ammonium nitrate and water in divided compartments in a special plastic bag. They have a long shelf life, do not need refrigeration, and can also be used outdoors. When using this bag, the bag is squeezed, which mixes the contents, which then generates cold temperatures by a chemical reac-tion.

Icepacks can be made with Ziploc bags filled with water and frozen in the freezer and then applied to the affected area. The duration of application for icepacks is about 20 to 30 minutes. A layer of towels can be applied between the icepack and the affected area. If Ziploc bags are unavailable, use a bag of frozen peas or other frozen vegetable from the freezer and wrap the frozen bag with towels, then apply it to the affected area.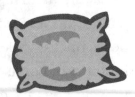

Ice Massage

Ice is applied in a massaging manner over the af-fected areas such as the elbows for conditions such as tendonitis. For this technique, use ice cubes from a re-frigerator at home. Sometimes, holding an ice cube can be difficult and slippery. A simple technique is to fill disposable paper cups with water and then freeze and use the frozen water cups by peeling the rim off the cup. In ice massage, the therapeutic effects of both ice and massage are used. The recommended duration for application of the ice massage is 5 to 10 minutes.

Pneumatic Compression/Cryotherapy Units

These units are used after total knee replacement. They have special cuffs in which cool water circulates through the cuff and helps relive acute musculoskeletal pain. These units also apply pneumatic compression. Here, the effects of pneumatic compression are also used to relieve pain in the affected area.

Vapocoolant Spray

Vapocoolant sprays containing fluoro-methane are sprayed on the affected area and are useful in muscle sprains. Vapocoolant sprays can be used prior to stretching sore muscles.

Contrast Baths

In contrast baths, the affected area of the body, usually an extremity such as the hands or feet, is immersed and alternated between hot and cold water for few minutes. The contrast of hot–cold creates a pumping action of the blood vessels and helps circulate the blood in the affected body part. The blood vessels dilate with heat and constrict with cold. Any stagnating swelling is reduced as it is pumped out of the body part. Inflammation is reduced as fresh blood and healing agents are pumped into the injured area. Pain is also reduced, as both hot and cold have anesthetic effects. This technique is useful in Complex Regional Pain Syndrome (CRPS) also called Reflex Sympathetic Dystrophy (RSD), carpal tunnel syndrome, tendonitis, and arthritis of the hands and feet.

Aquatic Physical Therapy

Aquatic physical therapy is similar to conventional physical therapy except that it occurs in a heated pool of water under the supervision of a physical therapist. Water supports the body and reduces stress to the joints to strengthen and tone muscles while injuries heal. Early joint movement is possible in water, even if the patient is experiencing pain. Aquatic physical therapy can be performed at various depths and can increase circulation, strength and endurance, range of motion, balance and coordination, and muscle tone. Aquatic physical therapy also protects joints during exercise. Only certain physical therapy clinics have aquatic physical therapy, so patients should check with local physical therapy centers. A water-heated pool is a good alternative to have at home to perform stretching and strengthening exercises.

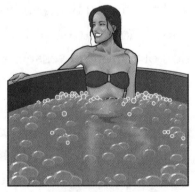

Iontophoresis

Iontophoresis is a means of delivering medication through the skin under the influence of electric current. The medication is applied to the skin, and then an electrical current is applied through special plates. The electric current causes the medication to migrate under the skin. Many different medications can be delivered in this fashion. One of the most common medications used is a steroid. Steroids produce an anti-inflammatory effect in the general area causing pain. This modality is especially effective in relieving acute episodes of pain. This is one approach for patients who cannot tolerate oral medications.

Phonophoresis

Phonophoresis is a method of delivering locally applied medications through the skin using ultrasound. Hydrocortisone and/or local anesthetic are mixed with a coupling jelly, and this mixture is applied to the affected area. Ultrasound is used at the same time, and the energy of the ultrasound drives the steroid particles into the affected area. Phonophoresis is useful in arthritis, bursitis, capsulitis, and tendonitis. Published clinical reports are available that show the efficacy of phonophoresis in bursitis of the shoulder.

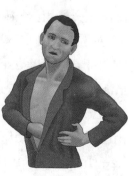

Electric Stimulation

Electrical current is used in two devices. A first device called transcutaneous electrical nerve stimulator (TENS) unit uses electrical stimulation to modulate the sensation in a painful area of the body such as the low back by preferential stimulation of certain nerve fibers (called A-beta fibers), which override the painful signals sent to the brain via the C- and A-delta fibers. A trial is usually performed first in a physical therapy center and, if the patient experiences substantial pain relief, a TENS unit may be used at home for chronic relief on a long-term basis.

A portable TENS unit resembles a pager (beeper), which is worn with a belt clip, and the extensions from the unit are applied with sticky electrodes similar to the cardiogram leads, though much smaller. The whole device can be concealed under clothing and provides continuous pain relief. There are patients with chronic pain who use such devices and go to work with these units. TENS is useful for neuropathic pain, which is nerve-related pain, and in chronic pain secondary to fibromyalgia and chronic myofascial pain.

A second device, a functional electric stimulation (FES) unit, is used to develop, strengthen, and stimulate weak muscles that cannot be strengthened by conventional physical therapy, especially in spinal cord injury. The idea of strengthening the muscles is to stabilize the joints and prevent chronic pain.

Traction

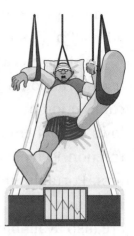

Traction is a technique in which pulling forces are applied to stretch a segment of the spine. This method is used for chronic neck and low back pain. Traction is known to relieve the compression on the nerves in the spinal segment of the neck and low back.

Cervical traction (traction to the neck) is applied with a chin sling called a Sayre Sling. Forces between 10 to 25 pounds are used to cause clinical effects of pain relief.

Lumbar Traction

Special traction tables are used and, with forces of about 80 to 150 lbs traction, are applied to the lumbar spine through special belts, which relieve pressure upon the nerves of the lumbar spine. Typical sessions involve 3 to 6 seconds of traction with a minute's rest after the traction. Such cycles continue for 30 to 60 minutes and are repeated 2 to 3 times per week.

Traction is dangerous in spinal infection, spinal tumors, rheumatoid arthritis, and osteoporosis because the risk of fracture of the vertebrae at the weakened bone is possible. Cervical traction is risky in carotid and vertebral artery disease because of potential stroke with the procedure. Traction should be considered an adjunct modality for the management of chronic pain. A physical therapist should initially demonstrate the use of traction before the traction is used offsite. Cervical traction units are available for home use, which allows the patient to apply at his or her leisure. Lumbar traction is typically handled at physical therapy centers. Portable units for lumbar traction that incorporate pneumatic traction units in compact lumbar brace are also available. One such unit has shown to reduce the tension inside the disc in disc herniation.

Massage

Massage therapy is an ancient and, yet, popular method for a variety of painful musculoskeletal conditions. Massage is known to cause mobilization of fluids, muscular relaxation, and vascular changes. Massage can be useful to mobilize soft tissue, decrease spastic muscle tone and reduce swelling, and increase blood flow to the soft tissues. In many conditions such as pain and paralysis, the poor muscle contractions impede the fluid mobilization from the tissues causing stasis of fluid and swelling. Massage can substitute for muscle contractions to enhance the lymphatic drainage and decrease swelling. It is a myth that

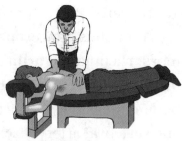

massage can improve and increase muscle strength; it cannot.

Massage therapy is risky in the following groups of patients: infection to the skin and soft tissues as there is a risk of spreading infection to the unaffected areas; cancer to the affected areas because the risk of spreading tumors to the unaffected areas; and areas of recent trauma because re-bleeding to the area is risky. One area of great caution: Massaging the calves, if there is an underlying blood clot as the clot can be dislodged into the lungs.

Orthotics (Splints/Braces)

An orthotic is a device attached to the external surface of the body to improve function, restrict or enforce motion, or support a body segment. Orthotics are important for pain control in patients with chronic pain. Splints, the prototype of orthotics, dates back to 2000 B.C. when the Egyptians used splints to hold an injured body part from further injury.

Soft Cervical Collar

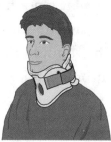

A soft collar is a foam pad that encircles the neck in a snug fit with Velcro straps. Soft collars are used for patients with minor neck sprains. A soft cervical collar does not restrict cervical motion, but provides warmth and psychological assurance and serves as a reminder to the wearer to hold the neck still.

Carpal Tunnel Splint

Patients with carpal tunnel syndrome have compression of the main nerve to the hand (median nerve) at the wrist from a variety of reasons including an old injury to the wrist. The median nerve compression is also dependant on the position of the wrist. The splint places the wrist in an optimum position and relieves pressure on the nerves of the wrist. Carpal tunnel splints are available over-the-counter and, in early cases, can be worn at night.

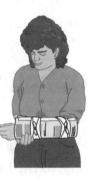

Patellar Tendon Bearing Brace

Ms. R.R. was a nurse who had a chronic, non-healing ankle injury from an old fracture. I prescribed a patellar tendon bearing brace for her, which, essentially, offloads the ankle by transferring the weight on the knee. This simple device gave Ms. R.R. a new life without chronic pain. A patellar tendon bearing brace is a good alternative for many painful conditions of the ankle and foot that are worse with weight bearing and for which the surgeon cannot perform further surgeries.

Tennis Elbow Splint (forearm bands)

Tennis elbow is a painful condition of the elbow caused by tendonitis of the muscles of the forearm. Patients have pain on the outer aspect of the elbow. The pain is not necessarily seen in tennis players, but also in individuals with repetitive use of their hands and forearms at home or work. Tennis elbow splint is a band that is applied to the forearm about an inch below the bend of the elbow. The purpose is to alleviate tension at the upper attachment of a key muscle of the forearm, which is responsible for tennis elbow.

Patella Stabilizing Brace

Patients with patello-femoral syndrome have constant pain in the front of their knees as a result of poor tracking of the patella (kneecap) in the grove of the thighbone (femur). The patella stabilizing brace acts to draw the kneecap toward the midline of the knee and prevents excess stress on the kneecap and the lower end of the thighbone and, thereby, reduces pain from patello-femoral syndrome.

Lumbar Corset/Brace

Lumbar corset use is controversial because using this brace can decrease the use of the muscles around the spine leading to weakening of these muscles, and lumbar braces are not recommend for chronic low back pain. Nevertheless, it is used temporarily in conditions such as acute back sprains, vertebral fracture, acute painful disc herniation, and following spine surgeries. These braces should be used only while standing and walking and should be removed while lying down. The idea of spinal exercise is to strengthen the muscles, which surround the spine, and protect it like a brace. Patients should always follow doctor's advice regarding this brace.

Exercises

Why do it: Patients do not like the idea of exercise when they are in pain, and it is the last thing they want to do. Most often, they go for one session and then do not want to continue because "it hurts." The skeletal system, with its contiguous muscles, ligaments, and tendons, is a "lever system" designed to carry weight; however, a poorly mobile joint or a weak muscle in the lever system can place undue stress on the lever system, which causes worsening pain or can perpetuate a painful state. For example, a tight hamstring can cause poor pelvic motion exacerbating low back pain. Weak biceps can cause pain in the arm after lifting unaccustomed weights.

Exercise in spinal disorders or other joints should be performed after spinal injections or joint injections because steroid-local anesthetic injections offer pain relief to continue exercise. Exercise induces the body to release special chemicals called endorphins, which actually block pain signals from reaching the brain. These chemicals also help alleviate anxiety and depression, which are commonly associated with chronic pain. Exercises are necessary to rehabilitate the spine and joints and help alleviate pain. Importantly, a regular exercise routine provides patients with the means to help avoid recurrences of pain and helps reduce severity and duration of potential episodes of pain in the affected area.

Regular exercise also improves sleep and provides more energy to cope with pain, as insomnia can perpetuate chronic pain. Exercises can help patients lose weight, which reduces stress on the joints. When people fail to exercise, as in prolonged bed rest, they became deconditioned. Deconditioned muscles, bones, and joints can hamper rapid rehabilitation and perpetuate pre-existing chronic pain problems. Inactivity raises the risk of high blood pressure, high cholesterol, and diabetes; these problems increase the chance of heart attack or stroke.

How to do it: Three common types of exercises prescribed in physical therapy are stretching exercise, strengthening exercise, and aerobic exercises. There are specific exercises for low back pain, shoulder impingement syndrome, carpal tunnel syndrome, etc.

Stretching/Flexibility Exercises

These exercises help reduce joint stiffness and allow you to move more comfortably. They also prevent your muscles from shortening and tightening. Almost everyone can benefit from stretching the soft tissues—the muscles, ligaments, and tendons around the joint. It is best to do stretching exercises, first thing, every morning. Think of it as a protective regimen for the body. Stretching can reduce the risk of further injury. Additionally, increased flexibility of the neck, shoulders, and upper back may improve respiratory function.

Stretching is done by slowly moving a joint toward its end-range of motion. You should feel a gentle "pulling" sensation in the target muscle. Hold this position for 15 to 30 seconds and then re-peat 3 to 5 times. Do not stretch to the point of pain, and do not bounce, since this may cause injury to the muscle. The stretch should be smooth and not jerky and maintain normal breathing during the stretches.

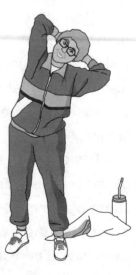

Avoid locking your joints while stretching the joints. Within a session, each subsequent stretch of a particular muscle group seems to give, progressively, more flexibility. Stretching should never hurt; therefore, limit your stretches to exclude pain. It may feel slightly uncomfortable, but should not be painful. Spend at least 20 minutes a day, three times a week doing stretching exercises. Start with your neck and progress to your shoulders, then the low back, hips, knees, and down to your feet.

If you've had a hip replacement, check with your doctor, as certain motions of the hip should be avoided after hip replacements. When combining stretching with another exercise such as aerobic exercise, stretches should be done after warm-up and cool down. Stretching is important after warm-up because it increases blood flow to the muscles. But stretching after cool-down may be even more important because stretching helps remove lactic acid from your muscles, which, in turn, reduces muscle soreness.

Common Recommended Stretches

Neck Stretch

Tilt your head forward as you press your chin in toward your chest. Hold for 15 to 30 seconds. Lift your head to return up to center, and then slowly tilt your head back by lifting your chin, and hold for 15 to 30 seconds. Inhale and gently bring your head back up to center. Next, allow your head to stretch to the right side by lowering your right ear toward your right shoulder and hold for 15 to 30 seconds. Feel the stretch along the left side of your neck. Similarly, repeat the stretch for the right side of your neck.

Shoulder Stretch (front)

Place flat palm of your right arm against a wall. Slowly rotate forward until you feel the stretch in your chest. Hold the stretch for 10 to 30 seconds. Stretch the other side.

Shoulder Stretch (back)

Extend your right arm in front of your body. Grab the right wrist with your left hand and pull the right arm inward toward your body, while keeping the right elbow extended. Hold for 10 to 30 seconds. Stretch the other side.

Triceps Stretch

Raise your right arm straight overhead, and then bend it behind your head toward your left shoulder blade. Grabbing your right elbow with your left hand, gently pull the right elbow toward your left shoulder to increase the stretch. Hold for 20 seconds, and then repeat with your left arm.

Forearm Stretch

Extend your right arm. Using your left hand, pull your fingertips back toward your body until you feel the stretch in your forearm. Hold the stretch for 10 to 30 seconds. Repeat using your other arm.

Cat Stretch (midback)

This exercise is to stretch your upper back. Place your hands and knees on the floor, just as a cat would do, then slowly lift your back up toward the ceiling and hold in place for 10 to 30 seconds.

Piriformis Stretch

Sit on a chair and bring your right ankle on top of your left knee. Grab your right knee with both hands and pull toward your chest. A stretch is felt in the right buttock area. Hold 20 seconds and relax.

Hamstring Stretch

The hamstring muscles seem to play a key role in low back pain. Tight hamstrings are common in back pain and stretching the hamstring muscles helps decrease the intensity of this pain and the frequency of recurrences. The hamstring muscle may be stretched in a number of different ways. The common methods for hamstring stretches are as follows:

Standing-Finger Tips–Toe Touch

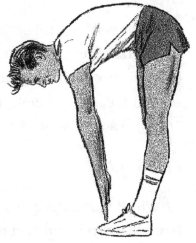

Bend forward at the waist, with your legs relatively straight, and try to touch your toes and hold this position.

Sitting-Finger Tips–Toe Touch

If the above approach is not well tolerated, sit on a chair and place your legs straight out in front on another chair, then reach forward and try to touch your toes. One leg at a time may be stretched.

Lie on the floor and loop a towel around the arch of one foot, while holding the ends of the towel. Pull this leg up and straighten by holding onto the towel that is wrapped behind the foot. One leg at a time may be stretched.

Quadriceps Stretch

While standing, hold onto a countertop or wall for balance, raise your right heel behind you, and take hold of it with your right hand or a looped belt. Pull your right foot toward your buttocks until you feel a gentle stretch on the front of your thigh. Hold for 20 to 30 seconds. Lower your right leg and repeat on the left.

Groin Stretch

While seated, pull both feet inward toward your body. Grab your feet with your hands, while using your elbows to press downward slightly on your knees. You should feel this stretch in your inner thighs. Hold for 10 to 30 seconds.

Calf Stretch

While standing, place your left foot near the wall. Bend forearms and rest them against the wall. Keeping the right foot flat on the floor, move your right leg back until you feel the stretch in your right calf muscle. Hold an easy stretch for 10 to 30 seconds. Do not bounce. Stretch the other leg.

Strengthening Exercises

Strength training increases your muscle mass and makes you stronger. Muscles by contracting burn excess fat. This helps you maintain a healthy weight, and muscle strength gained is important for rehabilitating sore joints. Strengthening exercises fortify the muscles around the joint, thereby acting as a brace around the sore joint, and take the load off bones and cartilage.

For example, building up your leg muscles with strength training can provide a natural brace for an arthritic knee. Strengthening the abdominal muscles, muscles around the spine and pelvic muscles, can support the spine like a brace. Muscle hypertrophy takes 2 to 4 weeks to start, so be patient if you do not see an increase in the size of your muscles.

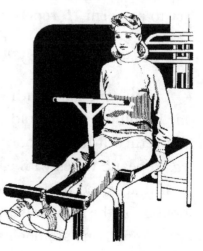

There is a big list of exercises for each of the muscles in the body. Some of the commonly recommended exercises are listed below. Remember there are several variations of the same exercise.

Ankle Pumps (lying on your back)

Lie on your back. Move your foot at the ankle up and down. Repeat 10 times. This will strengthen the muscles on the front and back of your leg.

Heel Slides (lying on your back)

Lie on your back. Slowly bend and straighten your knee. Repeat 10 times. This exercise will strengthen the quads and the hamstrings.

Pelvic Tilt Exercise (lying on your back)

Lie on your back with your knees bent. In this relaxed position, the small of your back should not be touching the floor. Tighten your abdominal muscles and roll your pelvis up so that your upper back presses flat against the floor. Hold for 5 seconds and then relax. Try to perform 10 repetitions.

Leg Raises (lying on your back)

Lie on your back with your arms at your sides. Lift one leg off the floor. Hold your leg up for a count of 10 and return it to the floor. Do the same with the other leg. Repeat 5 times with each leg.

If that is too difficult, keep one knee bent and the foot flat on the ground while raising your leg. This exercise strengthens stomach and hip muscles.

Partial Sit-Ups (lying on your back)

Lie on your back with knees bent and feet flat on the floor. Keep your hands on either side of the head.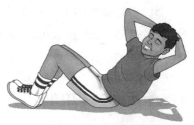

Slowly raise your head and shoulders off the floor halfway to sitting position. Count to 10 and then repeat 5 times. This exercise strengthens the muscles around your stomach.

Bird-Dog Exercise (on all fours)

This exercise strengthens the back muscles. Begin on hands and knees. Slowly lift one arm and the opposite leg off the floor. Hold briefly. Repeat with other arm/leg set. Do 10 to 20 repetitions.

If this is too easy, you can add weights to the wrists and ankles. Be sure to keep your neck in a neutral position (eyes looking at the floor).

Wall Squats (standing)

Stand with your back leaning against the wall. Walk 12 inches in front of your body. Keep abdominal muscles tight while slowly bending both knees 45 degrees. Hold 5 seconds.

Slowly return to upright position. Repeat 10 times. This exercise strengthens the back, hip, and leg muscles.

Heel Raises (standing)

Stand against the wall with your weight evenly distributed on both feet. Slowly raise heels up and down. Repeat 10 times.

Leg Raises (sitting)

You can also sit upright in a chair with legs straight and extended at an angle to the floor. Lift one leg waist high. Slowly return your leg to the floor. Do the same with the other leg. Repeat 5 times with each leg.

Swiss Ball Exercises

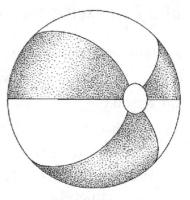

The Swiss ball is a large colored ball made of vinyl and inflated with air. Physical therapists in Sweden used the balls initially for rehabilitation of children with cerebral palsy. Subsequently, these balls were used for adults and, now, it is a commonly used equipment for exercise. Using a Swiss ball puts us in an unstable environment compared to a machine-based training program, and we are forcing ourselves to recruit our stabilizing musculature—particularly around our joints. The Swiss balls come in a variety of sizes. To determine the ideal size of the ball you should use, sit on the top of the ball and your thighs should be parallel to the ground. Use the following exercises with Swiss ball.

Walking the Ball with the Legs

Lie on your back on the floor with knees bent and calves resting on the ball. Slowly raise one arm overhead and then lower that arm, alternating right and left sides. Slowly straighten one knee and relax, alternating right and left sides. Slowly straighten one knee and rise opposite arm over head. Alternate opposite arms and legs. Slowly "walk" the ball forward and backward with your legs.

Stationary Marching

Sit on the ball with your hips and knees bent 90 degrees and feet resting on the floor. Slowly raise one arm overhead and lower that arm, alternating right and left sides. Slowly raise and lower heel, alternating right and left sides. Slowly raise one heel and rise opposite arm overhead. Alternate opposite arm and heel. Slowly raise one foot 2 inches from the floor, alternating right and left sides.

Lie with your stomach over the ball. Slowly raise alternate arms overhead. Slowly raise alternate legs 2 to 4 inches off the floor. Repeat above alternating opposite arms and legs. Be careful not to arch your low back.

Resistance Band

A resistance band is similar to a big rubber band and is available in different varieties of resistance. It can be tied to a firm support such as a doorknob with the other end held in your hand. It can be used in a wide variety of ways to strengthen the muscles of the upper limbs. Similarly, a resistance band can be attached to your foot to strengthen a number of muscles in your leg.

Wobble Board

Wobble board is a board with a small unstable base. It's used in the rehabilitation of chronic ankle injury to strengthen the muscles around the ankle. Patients with chronic ankle injury stand on these boards. As the name implies, the board is wobbly and, by trying to adjust the balance, a lot of muscles in the legs are strengthened. It can also help rehabilitate chronic ankle injury.

Endurance Exercises

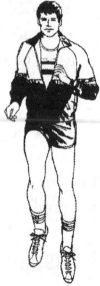

Endurance exercise (aerobic exercise) is the ability to perform cardiovascular exercises such as running, swimming, or brisk walking for an extended period of time. Aerobic exercises challenge your heart, lungs, and muscles, increasing your heart rate, blood pressure, and need for oxygen. The purpose of endurance exercise is to make the heart and lungs work better with less effort. For an exercise to be aerobic, it should fulfill the following criteria.

- The exercise must use the large muscles of the arms or legs such as the gluteal muscles, hamstrings, biceps, deltoid, etc.
- The exercise must feel like moderate work with faster breathing and more heartbeats each minute.
- The exercise must be done regularly (at least three times each week).
- The exercise has to be continuous and last for at least 20 minutes (not including warm-up and cool-down).

These exercises help your body function more efficiently and reduce your risk of heart disease, high blood pressure, high cholesterol, and diabetes. A common complaint among rehabilitation of patients with chronic pain is "I am tired." The reason is limited endurance. Limited endurance can reduce the quality of life to being bed or wheelchair bound.

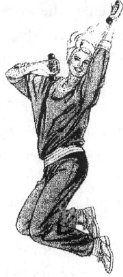

Aerobic activity increases your stamina so you aren't as easily fatigued during daily activities. These exercises improve sleep and mental health, reduce the effects of stress, and burn excess fat. Aerobic exercises maintain the spine in neutral position while stabilizing with abdominal muscles to protect the low back from future injuries.

Clinical studies have shown the efficacy of endurance exercises for a number of diseases; notable are fibromyalgia, diabetes, and congestive cardiac failure. Clinical studies have also shown mild-to-moderate intensity exercise training can result in cardiac changes similar to the effects induced by diuretics.

1. Where and What:

   Exercise should be tailored to your preferences. Choose one exercise or a combination of exercises.

   ♦   Swimming, stair-stepping, tread mill, and the stationary bike are also good endurance exercises.

   ♦   Get well-made equipment (e.g., walking shoes with good stability).

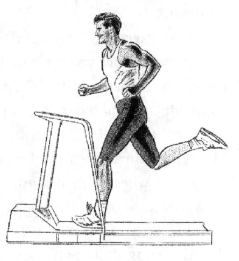

   Try to watch television or listen to your favorite music while working on a treadmill to enjoy the workout.

2. How Hard:

   ♦   Monitor your exercise intensity and duration.

   ♦   Start each session slowly and give yourself time to warm up (5 minutes).

   ♦   Judge how your body feels to help monitor exercise intensity.

   ♦   You should never be in pain or be unable to speak.

   ♦   Use the Rating of Perceived Exertion Scale (see below).

   ♦   Monitor heart rate (your doctor or physical therapist can help you with this).

- If you are on medications that affect your heart rate, talk to your doctor.
- Start slowly, but plan to work a little harder as weeks go by.

3. How Long:

- Duration may be 5 minutes at first, but plan to gradually increase.
- Progress to at least 20 minutes of continuous exercise each day.
- 30 to 45 minutes is ideal.

4. How Often:

Three to five days each week (do strengthening exercises on other days).

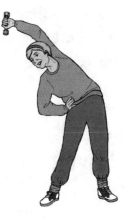

- If you do endurance exercise daily, alternate weight bearing with non-weight-bearing (i.e., walk one day, then ride or swim the next).

5. Safety:

- Be cautious if you start endurance exercise without professional guidance.
- Consider exercising with a partner or in a supervised facility.
- Consider seeing your doctor and an exercise professional before starting your endurance exercise program.

Be sure to drink liquids when you are exercising. If your doctor has asked you to limit your fluids, be sure to check with him or her before increasing the amount of fluid you drink while exercising. Congestive heart failure and kidney disease are examples of chronic diseases that often require fluid restriction.

Borg Scale for Perception of Exertion

This is a subjective measure of the level of exertion. This is a 15-point scale similar to the visual analog scale for pain. The scale starts at point 6 and ends at 20. Point 6 on the scale is the equivalent of sitting down doing nothing, point 9 on the scale is similar to walking gently, point 13 on the scale is a steady exercising pace, and 19 and 20 are the hardest exercises you have ever done. A desired Borg scale of perception of exertion during endurance exercise is 12 to 14.

Having Fun with Exercise

Endurance exercises with treadmills or stationary bikes can sometimes feel like a chore. Maybe you purchased one of those "exercise machines" and it's gathering dust. Try something different. The idea of exercise is to maintain good health and keep you fit. Activites can be a source of fun and, yet, are great exercises. (As a word of caution, talk to your doctor before trying these suggested exerecises).

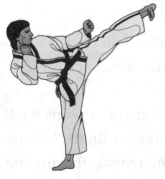

I suggest brisk walking, jogging, running, baton twirling,

bike riding, roller-skating, skate-
boarding, jumping rope, playing tennis (hitting tennis balls against a wall
if you cannot find a partner), squash,
racquetball, badminton, ping-pong,
riding or training horses, golfing (no
cart), rowing, diving, dancing (try
learning new moves), basketball,
baseball/softball, volleyball, football,
soccer, fencing, gymnastics, cheer-
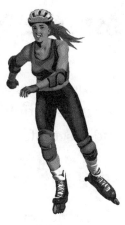
leading, martial arts, wrestling, water polo, field hockey,
ice hockey, and/or ice-skating.

If you like to stay around the house, there are lots of
things you can do such as chopping wood, mowing the
lawn, active gardening, scrubbing floors and/or win-
dows, housework, raking leaves, and shoveling snow.
For those who love outdoors, consider canoeing,
kayaking, rafting, sailing, walking, hiking, backpack-
ing, active bird watching, nature photography, moun-
tain climbing, and skiing. The list goes on. The bottom
line is: Think of exercise to maintain your health and
fitness and enjoy every
moment of it.

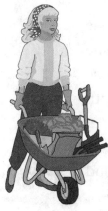

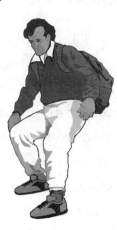

Assistive Devices for Chronic Pain

There are a lot of devices that can assist you in your activities of daily living and ambulation with less pain and discomfort. Review the following examples.

Cane

A cane is used for pain in the knee, hip, or unsteady leg secondary to sciatic symptoms. A cane increases the base of support and can take the weight off the affected limb by 25% of the body weight and give more balance with walking. Use the cane on the unaffected side, especially for painful hips. However, for painful knees, either side is acceptable. Do not use just any cane. The ideal height of the cane should reach approximately to the level of the hip.

Quad Cane

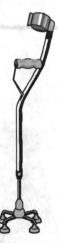

This is a cane with four prongs on the base. The advantage is that the quad cane stays upright, even if you momentarily lose your grip, which is common in patients with associated arthritis in the hands or carpal tunnel syndrome, where numbness or weakness in the hands can prevent a good grip on the cane.

Walker

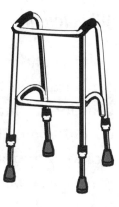

Use a walker when your gait is un-steady and a cane does not provide adequate support as in Parkinson's disease and associated stroke. A roll-ing walker has wheels for individuals who have problems with strength in lifting the walker while walking.

Axillary Crutch

An axillary crutch is used to off-load a limb (allows transfer of 80% of the body weight) and is useful for painful limbs sec-ondary to acute arthritis, chronic pain in the legs (worse with weight bearing), and/ or sprains in the ankle and knee joints. The top of the crutch should lie against the ribs, two to three finger widths from

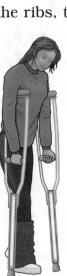

the armpit. The handgrips should be posi-tioned so there is a slight bend in the elbows. Never hang or press down on the underarm pads. All weight should be on the hands pressing against the handgrips. When as-cending stairs with crutches, climb one step with the good leg and then one step with the painful leg and crutch. When descending stairs, descend one step with the crutch and painful leg first and then with the good leg.

Wheelchair

Ambulation with the feet cannot always be a functional goal for all individuals with chronic pain. In such situations, ambulation using a wheelchair becomes a functional goal. A wide variety of

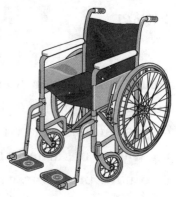

wheelchairs are available. Consult with your therapist and/or rehab specialist for the ideal wheelchair.

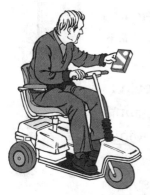

Reacher

The reacher is a commonly used device to grasp overhead objects, designed specifically for individuals with shoulder problems that limit full movement of the shoulder. Similarly, a reacher can be useful for individuals with poor spine and hip movement to lift objects on the ground.

Power Grip

This device can grip to jar caps and bottle caps and was designed for individuals with limited hand and finger strength, secondary to chronic arthritis, when pain limits opening jars and medication bottle caps.

Conclusion

Physical therapy and rehabilitation is one of the important facets in the multidisciplinary approach for the care of patients with chronic pain. The methods for physical therapy and rehabilitation are numerous, as outlined above, and they are effective in reconditioning after an injury. Rehabilitation methods through exercise and the adaptive devices described above are equally important, as the whole idea of pain management is not only lessening pain, but also improving function.

Notes

Chapter Seven

Cancer Pain Management and End of Life Care

Peter Kechejian, MD

Peter A. Kechejian, M.D. is an Interventional Pain Specialist and Director of Oncology Pain Services for North American Partners in Pain Management. A graduate of Georgetown School of Medicine, he completed his residency in Anesthesiology and fellowship in Pain Management at the University of Massachusetts Medical Center. Dr. Kechejian is a diplomate of the American Board of Anesthesiology with a Subspecialty Certification in Pain Management. He is formerly the Director of the Anesthesiology Pain Management Program at the Nassau University Medical Center on Long Island. He is a member of the International Spinal Injection Society and The New York State Society of Anesthesiologists.

Cancer Pain Management

Introduction

As many as 75% of all cancer patients have moderate to severe pain before they die. It is this very pain that most cancer patients fear the most when they are diagnosed and treated for their disease. With more aggressive pain management strategies, the percentage of patients who suffer from excessive pain can be reduced. Both from a moral and a medical model perspective, these patients should not feel that they will die with tremendous pain and suffering or feel they need to accept that uncontrolled discomfort is "part" of the dying process. Every patient has the right to receive the best pain care evaluation and treatment plan possible.

Not every patient talks about pain and copes with pain the same way. Oncologists do an excellent job treating a lot of the medical pain management that cancer patients need. In fact, 90% of pain can be managed quite effectively for most clinical cases, from the time of diagnosis until the end of life. It is the 10% of remaining patients who need a more aggressive, interventional pain management technique—that pain specialists typically get involved with—to get patients under better control at that point in their life.

More and more oncologists are encouraged to make appropriate referrals for advanced pain management evaluation when they are struggling to control a patient's symptoms. Interventional pain specialists are dedicated physicians who have mastered pain injection and implantable device techniques, such as nerve destruction or narcotic spinal pain pumps, to further treat intractable pain symptoms.

When looking at the extent of the problem, cancer deaths are second only to heart disease deaths. There are half a million new cases a year and half a million deaths annually from cancer. Severe unrelenting pain can lead to hopelessness and despair and becomes an essential focus of a cancer patient's life. It is this despair that dominates their lives and leads to terrible unnecessary suffering.

Certain types of cancer are associated with more pain than others. Metastatic cancer to bone is typically associated with the majority of pain that cancer patients feel. This severe bone cancer pain occurs in about 85% of patient cases. Oral cavity cancers have a lot of pain, in about 80% of the cases, and genitourinary cancers have about 75% pain issues. The least common cancer scenarios that cause pain are lymphomas and leukemias.

Who Is at Risk?

All patients who contract cancer are at risk of pain, but especially those cancer patients who suffer from metastatic bone disease, as described above. Virtually all of these patients can expect to have severe pain at some point in their course, if they are not adequately treated. The destruction of bone from spreading cancer needs heightened medical attention, so patients can receive appropriate and aggressive palliative treatment moving forward with their care. It is at this point in cancer pain care that patients move from a comprehensive medical pain management program, alone, to a program that includes interventional pain management techniques to get symptoms under control.

More patients need to take an active role in communicating their pain management needs to their primary physician and oncologists, so they receive timely and comprehensive pain care. If patients and their physicians are not aware of interventional pain relieving techniques, then they suffer the risk of continued pain under treatment as their disease progresses.

Our pain management group gives monthly lectures and presentations to physicians and the general public to educate them in the indications and advantages of interventional pain techniques. Falling short of the best pain management care available puts patients at risk of not only uncontrolled pain itself, but also the consequences of this severe pain, including anxiety, hostility, loneliness, depression, problems sleeping, and so forth.

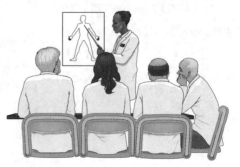

Causes of Cancer Pain

The most common cause of cancer pain is direct tumor involvement in either bone or around nerves. Another cause of cancer pain occurs when cancer attacks one of the organs in the body such as the pancreas. Intestinal obstruction can also be involved with direct tumor involvement. Direct tumor involvement accounts for about 78% of the causes of cancer pain. Another 19% can be caused by the cancer treatment itself. Only 3% of cases involve patients who have co-existing disease or disease states that exist in the body, separate from the actual cancer pain.

These co-existing pain states can be degenerative disc disease or osteoporosis, neuropathies in the body, or even muscular spasm pains. All potential pain sources need to be addressed so that no major pain area is missed or under treated. What real good would be served if the actual cancer-related pain were minimal and the patient were suffering from chronic sciatica from herniated discs? The point is that the "whole" patient needs treatment to get the best overall care effect, both physically and psychologically (anxiety and depression).

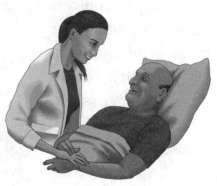

Types of Pain

A common type of pain arises from the musculoskeletal system and can be considered "somatic" pain. Metastatic cancer involving bones is a classic example of this type of pain and is often felt as dull and aching in nature. "Visceral" pain, or body organ pain, is another common type of pain. This type of pain is a dull, poorly localized ache that can be felt in another point in the body away from its original source. For example, pancreatic cancer can result in severe abdominal pain, as well as severe radiating back pain.

"Neurogenic" pain is another type of pain that arises from nerves, either from the spinal nerves or from peripheral nerves (example, sciatic nerve) in the body. This type of pain is often sharp, shooting, and electric in nature that typically radiates pain wherever the nerve or nerves travel in the body. There is also a category of psychological pain. If patients experience uncontrolled anxiety and depression, this type of psychological pain will be a problem, in and of itself, and can exacerbate the very real physical pain that patients experience.

When doctors discover where particular pains exist in their patients, it is at that point that medications and other treatments can be modified to best treat that specific type of pain. For example, bone pain responds better to traditional doses of narcotics than pain coming from nerves. It typically takes various anti-nerve medications, which are discussed later in this chapter, or very high doses of narcotics to get nerve-related pain under better control.

Management of Pain

The management of cancer pain follows three basic approaches. First, we need to eliminate the source of the cancer pain through primary treatment. This is primarily in the hands of the oncologist. Second, we need to treat the pain itself. Remember, the pain that cancer causes needs to be thought of as a "disease," itself, that needs full medical attention and care, so the painful process is fully treated. Third, we need to do combinations of the above two treatment approaches as care moves forward. By actively following these three methods of care, the oncology and pain management teams can achieve the best overall outcome of comfort for patients. It is this multidisciplinary team of oncologist, pain specialist, and any other involved health personnel that makes it possible for patients to receive the "standard of care" for their pain management.

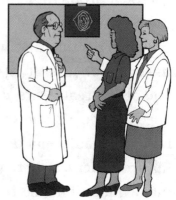

Anti-cancer pain treatment typically consists of surgical techniques to remove tumors, chemotherapy techniques, and radiation techniques. Surgical and medical oncologists direct these variations of cancer treatment. It is beyond the scope of this book to get into the details of specific surgical, chemotherapeutic, and radiological treatments available for cancer care. Discussions of various treatment options, depending on the cancer diagnosis, are best left to the medical and surgical oncologists. Cancer care is an incredibly complex area of medicine and it behooves patients to seek out a cancer team that will take the time to listen to their concerns and issues and develop a reasonable treatment plan moving forward with care.

The use of oral and intravenous narcotics is important to treat cancer pain as it occurs. These are considered the standard of medical pain management. These narcotics are of many types and are strong enough to control different intensities of pain. Anti-inflammatory medications, antidepressants (to help with mood and pain), muscle relaxants, and so forth are all additional medications that work with narcotics to help control different types of pain (sharp pain, electric pain, spasm pain, etc.). Spinal narcotics can be used in more advanced cases, either through an epidural injection or intrathecal (spinal fluid) injection. Neurosurgical techniques are not very common, but in very advanced, severe cases, lesioning the spinal cord itself, called cordotomy, can lead to some pain relief, especially in patients whose life expectancy is only a few weeks or months.

A TENS unit, physical therapy, acupuncture, and treatments along this course are also used to manage pain through a non-medication approach. Behavioral therapies are also included in the multidisciplinary approach to overall comprehensive care. The chief advantage of narcotics is that they are the most effective as potent painkillers because they alter the perception of pain in addition to changing the patient's "reaction" to pain. A kind of euphoria a patient can feel with the use of potent narcotics can make them indifferent to the physical and psychological stressors associated with their disease. This is an excellent effect for actively dying patients at the end of their life. We will talk more about end-of-life care at the end of this chapter.

Pharmacological Therapies

The World Health Organization and other pain management organizations developed an analgesic stepladder approach to help doctors and nurses better treat pain of both an acute and cancer pain nature. Agony should be considered an emergency and needs to be evaluated as promptly as possible. There are several important principles that health professionals should realize while treating pain patients. Treating personnel should not underestimate the effective dose of narcotics they use. In other words, physicians should know standard dosing of medications and when to increase doses of narcotics in already tolerant patients.

A second principle of treatment is not over-estimating the duration of action of these narcotics. A lot of physicians are prescribing narcotics on an every 4- to

6-hour basis when, in fact, the patient is only getting relief for 3 hours. In this case, the medication should be rewritten for every 3 hours, especially if the patient is not having any side effects to the narcotic.

A third principle is that health personnel should not exaggerate the addictive potential of strong narcotics, especially when dealing with palliative care cancer pain management. Even using strong narcotics such as morphine and Dilaudid in the acute postoperative setting for days to weeks is extremely unlikely to result in a patient becoming a drug addict once they leave the hospital. Patients who are in severe pain use strong narcotics as prescribed by their doctors to control the pain, not to get high.

Typically, when we start the stepladder approach to treat different intensities of pain, physicians start with non-narcotics such as aspirin or Tylenol or nonsteroidal anti-inflammatory medications such as ibuprofen or naproxen. These medications are excellent for the treatment of mild pains. Beyond this, we start moving to weak narcotics such as codeine or hydrocodone (Vicodin) or Oxycodone (Percocet). These narcotics are excellent for the treatment of moderate pains.

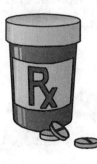

Moving further up the ladder, the next step is to use stronger narcotics if patients are experiencing severe pain. Morphine, Dilaudid, or the fentanyl patch (Duragesic) is the choice for treating pain at this level of high intensity. Beyond this, the fourth step involves the use of implantable spinal narcotic pump therapies or nerve destructive techniques. More information about these step-four techniques is discussed later in this chapter.

At all of these stepladder levels of primary pain medication usage, there are additional medications called adjuvant medications that can be helpful in managing patients along the way. Some of these medications include antidepressants (Elavil, Effexor), anti-anxiety medications (Xanax, Ativan, Valium), stimulants (Ritalin) for over sedated patients, anti-nausea medications (Compazine, Vistaril, Zofran), stool softeners (Senokot, Colace, Miralax), etc. By combining narcotics and adjuvant medications, patients can receive the best comprehensive medical pain available.

Reassessment at all levels is critical while treating cancer pain ensuring that we determine effective doses of pain management based on balancing relief with minimizing potential side effects. Excessive side effects of treatment should not be accepted as part of the medication process and, in fact, can cause more distress to patients than the pain itself. Constipation, nausea, and excessive sleepiness are all common potential side effects of narcotic usage that need to be actively addressed on a continuous basis. Adjuvant medications, as mentioned above,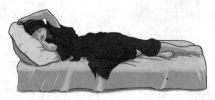

are typically necessary to combine
with narcotics to help with dose-
limiting side effects.

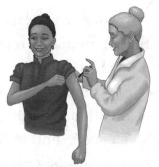

Several important guidelines
for optimizing narcotic use to
keep patients comfortable are
available. First, doctors and
nurses should administer narcotics on a time basis,
rather than on an as-needed basis, especially if patients are hurting constantly. Various long-acting narcotics such as the Duragesic fentanyl patch, MS Contin
long-acting morphine, Oxycontin, and methadone can
take care of this around-the-clock pain need quite effectively.

When a particular long-acting narcotic is trialed, patients will either achieve an acceptable level of comfort
or they will experience untoward side effects. If the excessive side effects come first, and are persistent despite treatment, then a different long-acting narcotic
should be trialed, and so forth.

A second guideline is to remember to provide adequate doses of medications using sedation or respiratory rate as an end point, again, to ensure patients receive adequate pain relief and not experience excessive
side effects. Doctors typically use a long-acting narcotic
agent that they are familiar with, so that they can be
comfortable with this, as they need to increase doses
accordingly. Increases in the dose are typically needed
as patients develop tolerance to medications. Developing tolerance is a normal process of using strong

narcotics, where more and more are needed through time to maintain a certain level of pain relief.

A third guideline is that it is important to remember to combine narcotics with the adjuvant medications, as mentioned earlier, to optimize therapy and minimize side effects, and always remember that potential drug dependency should not be a primary consideration in the cancer patient.

Spinal narcotics are used if patients remain in intractable pain, despite higher and higher doses of oral morphine or other narcotics, especially if the oral morphine doses approach more than 250 mg daily and/or if patients are experiencing intolerable side effects on their oral narcotic regimen such as over sedation, fatigue, loss of appetite, or nausea, etc.

Implantable spinal narcotic catheters are used if patients are expected to live well beyond 3 months. For patients who are not expected to live for 3 months, longer-term epidural catheter placement can be considered in appropriate patients. A longer duration of life expectancy has been associated with better pain control using the spinal fluid narcotic catheter. Also, the tendency to experience fewer side effects using the spinal route of administration, compared to oral and intravenous narcotics, makes the spinal narcotic catheter and pumps an especially attractive option.

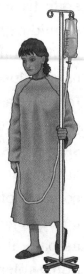

Nerve Blocking Techniques

The celiac plexus "alcohol" nerve block for stomach and pancreatic cancer can be very effective in reducing the patient's abdominal pain, especially if narcotics, themselves, are not adequately controlling the pain. These types of injections can be performed safely with patients under intravenous sedation and using an x-ray machine for accurate placement. A special medical preparation of alcohol is injected around nerves to keep them from sending painful impulses for up to 6 months. This duration of relief, which can be 75% or better, is typically long enough to keep patients comfortable until the end of their lives.

Another nerve-blocking technique involves using cryoanalgesia (nerve freezing technology) for metastatic bony rib pain. This method of pain control for severe rib pain is very effective. When patients are comfortably sedated under intravenous anesthesia and using the x-ray machine, a specialized probe is placed under each affected rib and, by freezing the nerve that controls the pain, these patients can get many, many weeks to months of relief.

Both the celiac plexus alcohol block and the cryoanalgesia procedures are excellent nerve blocking choices when more conservative therapies have failed to get adequate relief for patients. The best part of using these nerve injection procedures is that once better relief is obtained, these patients can lower their typically excessive narcotic load and start to have a better quality of life with less medication side effects.

Non-Pharmacologic Therapy

Non-pharmacologic therapy can consist of physical therapy techniques, behavioral techniques, acupuncture, TENS, and many other forms of adjuvant therapy to work with traditional pharmacologic agents and optimize the patient's comfort in a comprehensive multidisciplinary way. Physical therapy is important to maintain patient function as much as possible, so this adds to their quality of life and decreases disability. This helps patients maintain their "activities of daily living" such as walking, cooking, cleaning, and so forth.

Behavioral techniques such as bio-feedback, relaxation, hypnosis, or guided imagery are all very important to help patients cope with their very difficult problem. Specialists are available in all of these areas to work with patients both in the hospital and at home.

The TENS (transelectrical nerve stimulator) unit can be used, again, to help with regional pain, using mild electrical impulses to help block the pain impulses in that area. The TENS unit can work on pain in the arms and legs, as well as the back and chest. Patients should always focus on obtaining the best pain control possible while continuing to maintain as much function in their lives, based on the severity of each individual's disease process.

End of Life Care

End-of-life care is a particularly important aspect of pain management, especially when patients are expected to live for only a week or two. Emotional support to the patient and their family is also important, as well as continuing the aggressive pain management techniques they were using earlier in their course. Patients need to have their end of life wishes known, and many of them will sign advanced directives and do-not-resuscitate orders, so they do not get medical therapy that prolongs their life but, rather, make them quite uncomfortable at that time.

Special attention to excessive anxiety and depression needs to be taken care of, as well as optimizing their pain management regimen. In their final few weeks, many patients may require a continuous morphine infusion for their comfort with aggressive titration based on their clinical course. This morphine infusion can be administered while the patient is in the hospital or it can be arranged for a home pain care setting. Many health care personnel understand that it is okay to allow patients to make the decision to use more and more narcotics as pain increases, and realize that the increased pain medication helps their end-of-life pain, but may also speed up their eventual demise.

In moral principles, this is known as the "double effect," again, where more aggressive attempts to use narcotics at the end of life help pain, but, again, hasten their death. When used this way, for terminally ill patients, effective methods of pain control have nothing to do with physician-assisted suicide and everything to do with excellent end-of-life pain care. Patients may experience a number of different symptoms at the end of their life, besides the pain itself, and these need to be treated aggressively. Many patients may demonstrate muscle jerks and these can be treated with muscle relaxing medications such as like Ativan or thorazine, for example.

Many patients are in a hospital setting at the end of their life and receive narcotics intravenously by a patient-controlled analgesic pump (IV-PCA), with a continuous infusion and a dose given over a certain time, as the patient wishes. Some patients move toward a hospice outpatient setting where a hospice care network can care for their multidisciplinary needs in an outpatient setting, so they are comfortable at home for the remainder of their life. Whatever the setting, it is important that all health personnel follow this end-of-life sequence of patient care for the betterment of the patient, as well as the other people involved, especially family.

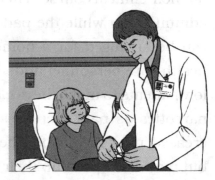

Case Example

A 45-year-old male is recently diagnosed with metastatic pancreatic cancer and is having severe abdominal pain radiating to his back. This patient was following his oncologist's regimen of cancer care, but having episodes of "9/10" abdominal pain, despite being on Percocet medication. The patient was taken to the hospital and placed on an intravenous morphine patient-controlled pump to try and get better control of this patient's pain. He was extremely nauseous and over sedated on increasing doses of morphine.

The oncologist had the pain management specialist evaluate the patient, and it was determined that a nerve block, specifically a celiac plexus alcohol nerve block, could be performed in a palliative care fashion to try and help this patient's severe pain. The risks and benefits of the celiac plexus block were explained to the patient and his family and everyone decided it was the best course of action at that time.

The patient had this neurolytic nerve injection performed successfully under intravenous sedation and x-ray guidance with 75% pain relief of his abdominal pain. The patient was able to decrease his narcotic need and his appetite improved 24 hours after the injection. He was less sedated and started to interact more with the people who came in contact with him. He could control his life more fully and this was a huge quality of life concern. It was noted that the patient's family was also delighted that the patient had better control of his pain and could function better with them. The patient eventually moved to a hospice setting where he was comfortably controlled, back on an oral medication, to the end of his life.

This case example illustrates several important points about cancer pain management. Given this patient's difficult aggressive diagnosis of pancreatic cancer, the oncologist offered all that was available in terms of primary cancer treatment therapy.

Because of the severe pain nature, the patient moved through an analgesic ladder of an oral narcotic to an intravenous narcotic and, eventually, needing a nerve block technique to get his intractable pain under control. This was successful in the end by combining both medical and interventional pain management. The patient had good end-of-life hospice care at home in a comfortable setting in a very meaningful and valuable way.

A Second Example

A 35-year-old female was diagnosed with breast cancer. She underwent primary cancer therapy and did well for 5 years in remission. One day, she started to experience increasing pain in her left leg that was, eventually, diagnosed as metastatic breast cancer disease. This news was devastating and, with the increasing pain that followed, she lapsed into a depression.

The patient failed to get relief with the increasing stepladder narcotic therapy approach, starting with

Motrin and Tylenol, moving up to Percocet and then, eventually, oral Dilaudid narcotic medication.

She had intolerable side effects of nausea and over sedation and still had "7/10" pain in her left thigh. She was evaluated by orthopedics and felt to be at risk for pathologic fracture. They suggested inserting a metal rod through the bone to stabilize the leg and keep it from fracturing. The patient agreed, and this was completed successfully in a palliative care fashion in a nearby hospital.

While the patient was recovering in the hospital after her surgery, the patient's oncologist consulted the pain management specialty team to evaluate her for eventual outpatient management. It was determined that this patient had been failing medical pain management (the first three stepladder pain management approaches) and was a candidate for the intrathecal (spinal) narcotic infusion pump. The spinal narcotic therapy could be started in the hospital and continued in the outpatient setting. This was discussed with the patient and her family and found to be favorable, realizing that the patient still had severe pain, despite high dose narcotics, and was still very drowsy.

The patient had a successful narcotic test trial while hospitalized with 2 mg of morphine placed in the spinal fluid space. The patient's pain reduced from "7/10" to "1/10" within half-an-hour and was not nauseous or over sedated. A day later, the permanent spinal narcotic pump was successfully placed without complication and doses were increased slowly. The patient was discharged from the hospital and, over the next month, the morphine pump was further increased to maintain the patient's comfort. The patient lived for two years in a very comfortable way, while she finished up her palliative care oncology treatment. She died comfortably at home surrounded by her family, again, in a meaningful and appreciative way.

This second case example illustrates, again, successful pain management moving through different stages of medical pain management and, eventually, to an interventional pain management technique such as the placement of spinal narcotic pumps. Pain management specialists are frequently called to evaluate patients for oncologists to help manage their patient's pain more aggressively, so they can continue with their ongoing cancer needs, moving forward.

The pain management team works in a meaningful way with the oncology team, in this fashion, to ensure that the patients do not experience uncontrolled pain or fear of dying with extreme pain. As oncologists become more and more aware of these situations, successful advanced pain management techniques can be offered in their area.

Oncologists will continue to call on pain specialists to be more involved in their patient's care as they battle their disease, especially for patients who cannot get comfortable with medical pain management alone. Many other case examples could be illustrated, but the above examples speak volumes for what can be accomplished in cancer pain management.

Conclusion

It is very important for patients to know that they do not have to fear dying with severe pain, especially when they are given a diagnosis of cancer. It is also important for the patients to realize that they should have "hope" as their cancer is treated. Patients should realize that the cancer disease process itself, needs to be treated foremost, maximizing options such as surgery, chemotherapy, and radiation. Treating the cancer aggressively makes treating the pain easier. Patients should understand that pain is invariably part of this difficult cancer process and needs to be aggressively attacked, as if it is a serious medical condition, in-and-of itself.

Following a medical pain management plan first, and then adding interventional techniques, as necessary, maximizes patient's comfort. The bad news of a palliative care diagnosis and treatment plan does not mean that patients are dying tomorrow, it just means there is no cure for their disease, at this time, based on current medical knowledge. Patients, in fact, can live for many, many years depending on how aggressive their cancer is and many other factors. Better control of intractable pain adds quality to life and often extends the duration of life itself. When it comes to caring for cancer patients, optimizing pain relief and their quality of life is the most important aspect of palliative care and end-of-life care.

Oncologists who need pain management specialty consultation should not fear losing patients to the pain management specialists. Our group's philosophy, for example, is to help an oncologist in any way with the management of their patients' pain, so the oncologists, themselves, can continue with the cancer care and not have uncontrolled pain as a major distraction. Many patients and their families are getting educated through books, public pain management presentations, and the Internet regarding the more advanced options of cancer pain management, should they need them. Patients need to continue to ask their doctors questions about their pain care, so they can make better-informed decisions. The major goal of all pain management is for patients to feel better and continue to live their lives. This philosophy of pain care should be shared with everyone.

Notes

Notes

Chapter Eight

How to Talk to Your Doctor About Pain

Mary Milano Carter, APRN, BC, MS

Mary Milano Carter, APRN, BC, MS is the Nurse Practitioner and Director of Clinical Services for North American Partners in Pain Management. She completed her Master of Science and Nurse Practitioner degrees at Adelphi University in Garden City, NY and has been a Registered Nurse for 17 years. She is Board Certified as an Adult Nurse Practitioner, Gerontological Nurse, and Medical-Surgical Nurse. She is the founding President of the American Society for Pain Management Nursing–Long Island Chapter and has been an active member of the American Society for Pain Management Nursing, the Oncology Nursing Society, The New York State Nurse Practitioner Association, and Sigma Theta Tau International Honor Society for Nursing for many years.

How to Talk to Your Doctor About Pain

Why is pain such a big deal in healthcare? The Joint Commission on Accreditation of Healthcare Organizations (JCAHO) recognizes pain as a major, but highly avoidable healthcare problem. The JCAHO is a national regulatory agency for hospitals and healthcare systems. The JCAHO, in conjunction with the University of Wisconsin, created new expectations for the assessment and management of pain in patients. The American Pain Society, a professional group that promotes pain treatment, education, and research, also endorses these standards. These new standards were implemented and hospitals are now expected to comply with them. This means that patients that are cared for by a hospital have the right to have their pain assessed, treated, and reevaluated. Staff must have the necessary education and competencies in place to care for patients in pain. Hospitals are graded by the JCAHO on an ongoing basis. If the grade is not good, the hospital can lose their accreditation.

Did you know that pain is the number one reason why people seek medical attention? Besides chest pain, which requires immediate attention, think about all the common conditions that can cause chronic pain such as cancer, stroke, migraine headaches, arthritis, diabetes, HIV and AIDS, surgery, trauma, accidents, and work related injuries; the list is endless! It seems that every disease state has the potential to cause pain. It is estimated that 75 million Americans suffer from pain at any given time with 50 million of those suffering from chronic pain.

Chronic pain is defined as any pain that lasts longer than three months. The National Institutes of Health recently assessed that chronic pain costs the U.S. economy 100 billion dollars annually in lost wages and pain treatment. With these numbers, it seems as if pain is a national health crisis. But many people do not like to see their healthcare providers and complain about what aches and pains. If you are suffering, it is important to tell your doctor quickly and provide as much information as you can about the pain. Pain is a signal from your body that something is wrong. This warning sign should not be ignored. Fast diagnosis and treatment is essential to prevent progression of disease and other problems that may occur. Would you know how to explain your pain to your doctor or nurse?

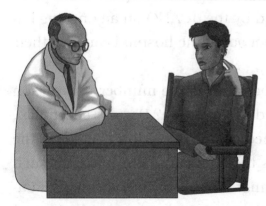

Start a Conversation

Usually, the first healthcare provider contact for a patient in pain is the primary care provider. It is important to provide as many details as you can about your pain, so you can be referred to the appropriate specialist(s) for treatment. You may need a further workup by an orthopedist, neurologist, neurosurgeon, rheumatologist, physiatrist, psychiatrist, psychologist, or an anesthesiologist who is also an interventional pain management specialist. You may even be referred to a physical therapist, licensed acupuncturist, chiropractor, or massage therapist. All of these other doctors and care givers will work with your primary care provider and each other to get your pain diagnosed and treated appropriately.

First

Chronic pain presents differently from acute pain (like pain from an incision after surgery or the pain of a fractured hip following a fall). Most acute pain sufferers wear their pain on their sleeves. They have high blood pressures and heart rates, may be sweating or rocking, or have facial grimacing. Chronic pain sufferers, in general, present much different than acute sufferers and appear normal in every way. It is sometimes hard for others to even believe that the person is, indeed, in pain because he or she "looks normal." Pain is not objective. There is no blood test, CAT scan, or blood pressure check to reveal that the patient is in pain. Pain is very subjective. Only you know how you feel.

Often, health care providers rely on numeric scales rating pain from zero (no pain) to 10 (the worst pain ever experienced). The same scale with visuals such as smiling and frowning faces that relate to the numbers are used for children and cognitively impaired adults.

This patient self-report of pain is the best tool providers have for basic assessment of chronic pain. The first piece of information your provider needs is your current pain score. Using a numeric or visual scale, rate your current pain level. It is also helpful to state your pain's highest score (your pain at its worst) and lowest (your pain at its best) score. With your pain scores, your doctor needs to know the aggravating activities (things that make your pain worse) and alleviating activities (things that ease your pain). These can be any activity including body positions such as sitting, standing, or laying down; physical activities such as walking, exercising, housework, or climbing stairs to usual pain relieving activities such as ice or heat application to the painful area, stretching, massage, or meditation.

Second

The second piece of information should describe when the pain started. Was there a cause? Some sufferers know the exact cause of their pain. It is chronic knee pain from osteoarthritis, menstrual migraines, chronic pain in the chest wall months after a mastectomy or open-heart surgery, or neck pain from a herniated disc following a motor vehicle accident. But some patients cannot actually pinpoint exactly what happened to start their pain. That is okay because the pain is still treatable! Most elderly folks with low back, neck, and joint pains suffer from arthritis and never even know that they have arthritis until they "wake up one morning" in pain. In a condition like arthritis, simple movement such as shutting off an alarm clock in the morning, lifting up a child, taking out the trash, or using a pooper-scooper can trigger pain! Knowing the cause of pain is beneficial because those activities can be avoided in the future. Not knowing the exact cause of pain places a lot of responsibility on the patient to exercise extreme care with all activities of daily living to avoid future pain episodes.

Third

In addition to discussing the cause of pain and how long it has occurred, the third piece of information is how the pain has changed over time. The pain of some conditions peak after onset and remain consistently painful, some peak and slowly ease off, while others peak and a new, more intense pain takes over. Use adjectives such as mild, discomforting, distressing, horrible, severe, and excruciating to describe how you have felt over time.

Describing your pain may be difficult. Pain can have different physical feelings, and it is different in every person. Pain can be sharp and shooting like electricity; it can burn like a flame; or be dull, achy, and constant like a toothache. These descriptions help your provider make a proper diagnosis of your pain.

Listening to the patient's complaint and taking a full history and physical examination enables the provider to make a diagnosis. You may be sent for radiological tests or blood work to confirm the diagnosis. Of course, the area of your body where the pain is located is usually one of the first things the patient mentions when conversing with a provider.

It is important to know if the pain radiates or travels to other parts of the body and if the pain feels differently in different areas of the body. Any other physical symptoms associated with your pain are important to communicate. These include any muscle weakness or spasm, loss of motion in a joint, new onset bowel or bladder incontinence (inability to retain urine or feces),

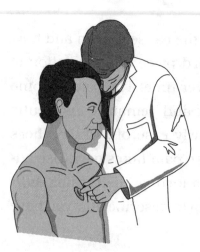

swelling in the painful area, or skin color or temperature changes. Other significant information includes any feelings of depression or anger, unexpected weight changes, or lack of physical activity.

Pain is generally a vicious cycle. Patients with

pain become more sedentary (inactive) because of the inability to work and play like they are accustomed to. Lack of physical activity creates depression and stress. Depression and psychological stress makes your pain worse and can decrease immune function. And, of course, weight gain or loss goes along with the depression. If pain and these other symptoms are not addressed, the patient is looking at other potential health problems. Experiencing chronic pain can subject the patients to loss of workdays or loss of job and can cause an economic hardship on the patients and their families. We break this vicious cycle by diagnosing the cause of pain, treating the disease and symptoms of pain, and using rehabilitation to return your life to normal—the lifestyle you are accustomed to living. Restoring the patient back to maximum function is the key!

Fourth

The fourth piece of information your provider needs to know is how you have dealt with the pain over time. This is especially important when you are seeing a specialist. You should keep your own records including a pain diary and copies of test results and reports. A pain diary is a written daily account, by you, that reflects how you feel each day. Include your pain level and activity level and if and how it changes. Was it a rainy day and you felt horrible? Did you go swimming and felt great afterwards? Also, include your mood and stress level.

Reading a pain diary, over time, can pinpoint patterns in pain and help with diagnosis and treatment. What other physicians and providers have you seen? What have they done for you, and did it work? What medications have you been taking or have taken in the past to help with the pain? This includes any prescription medications, any over-the-counter medications, and any vitamins or herbal supplements that you have tried. Quite frankly, any recreational drugs such as marijuana or prescription drugs purchased illegally on the street are also important facts to disclose. Even alcohol consumption for pain relief should be divulged. Of course, you need to report what worked or did not work for you and if you had any side effects. Remember, some side effects are normal and expected and are not considered an allergic reaction such as constipation from narcotic medications.

Fifth and Beyond

Every specialist you see should obtain your full medical and surgical history. All medical diagnoses need to be disclosed, as these are taken into consideration when discovering what is causing your pain. Since there are so many different disease states that can cause pain, as discussed earlier, your provider will consider every possible cause of your discomfort.

Your medical and surgical histories also influence medication selection. For example, certain medications commonly used to treat pain can interfere with other

medications you are already taking such as the blood thinner
warfarin. If you are taking warfarin, you are not a candidate to
take non-steroidal medications
such as ibuprofen due to increased risk of bleeding.

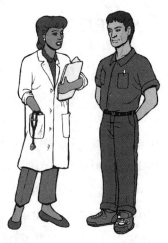

In addition, there are disease
states that may be worsened by
medications. For example, if you
suffer from extreme constipation, you may not be a
candidate for narcotic medications because constipation is one of the most reported side effects from these
medications. Any allergic reactions to any medications
or foods taken in the past should also be discussed.
Cross-allergies among medications are common. Some
food allergies (such as bananas, for example) may indicate other allergies such as a possible allergy to la-
tex, which is a common substance in hospitals and
doctor's offices.

Reactions to anesthesia from any previous surgeries should also be discussed. If you are a candidate for
interventional pain management (such as a nerve block),
intravenous anesthesia can be used to put you in a twi-
light sleep to numb the pain of the injection and help
you remain still and calm. If you have an allergy to eggs,
you cannot have a common intravenous amnestic called
propofol.

Furthermore

It seems that there is a lot of information to be shared with each provider you meet. But we are not done yet! Other helpful information includes discussing other immediate family members that suffer from chronic pain. Some painful medical conditions are hereditary. You should also inform your provider(s) of your occupation. Some things you do at work on a daily basis may be aggravating or contributing to your pain condition. Your job may have to be modified or changed in order for you to return to full function.

If your pain was caused by your job and you have a workman's compensation case pending, or if you have a lawsuit pending over an accident, notify your provider(s) immediately. Make available any contact names and addresses of your workman's compensation board or lawyer and do not forget to ask for a signed release authorizing your provider's office to send progress notes to those contacts, as well as your primary care provider. Current government regulations known as the Health Insurance Portability and Accountability Act, or HIPAA, requires a formal release signed by the patient because sending notes without this release is considered a breech of patient confidentiality.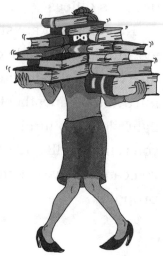

In Conclusion

It is very important to tell your provider about any pain you are experiencing. The faster you seek treatment, the faster you will feel better and return to your normal activities of daily living. Be an advocate or supporter for yourself. Speak up, describe your condition honestly and how it effects you and those around you. You can also use this information if you are advocating for a loved one that cannot speak for him/herself. Remember, complete pain relief may not be possible, but it can be decreased and controlled. Be prepared to make changes in your behavior, thinking, and lifestyle, and set goals for yourself.

Notes

Index

Notes

Notes

Notes